# The Suttons' Texts of 1916-1975

AND

ETIOLOGIC CLASSIFICATION OF DISEASES OF THE SKIN

# The Suttons' Texts of 1916-1975

## AND
## ETIOLOGIC CLASSIFICATION
## OF DISEASES OF THE SKIN

*By*

RICHARD L. SUTTON, JR., M.D., Sc.D., F.R.S.E.

Emeritus Clinical Professor of Medicine (Dermatology),
University of Kansas

Adjunct Professor in Medicine, Ophthalmology, and
Geosciences, University of Missouri-Kansas City

1981

KANSAS CITY, MISSOURI

**Library of Congress Cataloging in Publication Data**
Sutton, Richard Lightburn, Jr., 1908-
Etiologic classification of diseases of the skin.
Prefaces by Richard L. Sutton and Richard L Sutton, Jr.
Includes index.
1. Skin–Diseases–Etiology–Addresses, essays, lectures. 2. Dermatology–Classification–Addresses, essays, lectures. I. Sutton, Richard Lightburn, 1878-1952. II. Title. [DNLM: 1. Dermatology–Biobibliography. 2. Skin diseases–Classification. WR 15 S967e]
RL75.S87 616.5'0012 81-81915
ISBN 0-913504-68-8 ACCR2

Books available from the author at $17.50 per copy
3203 West 83rd Terrace, Leawood, Kansas 66206
and from The Lowell Press, Inc.
115 East 31st St., P.O. Box 1877, Kansas City, Mo. 64141–1877

# Contents and Index

# Foreword

Prefaces and title pages of nonmedical books of ours, portraits, and biographic data are included and should be of interest to librarians and readers with a historical bent.

A title page is standardly printed on the right, on a page of odd number, but for convenience here I put each on the left, where it identifies the preface next following.

Permission to reproduce previously published material was granted by the following publishers, whom I thank for their courtesy: Marquis Who's Who Inc.; Royal Society of Edinburgh, Year Book 1951/52 pp 45-48; The C. V. Mosby Company; Yorke Medical Books Division of Dun-Donnelly Publishing Corp., a company of Dun and Bradstreet Corp.

For their superior skill and cooperation in bringing the book off, I am grateful to Arthur Lowell and Barbara Funk, my publisher and editor.

# The Suttons' Texts of 1916-1975

## AND
## ETIOLOGIC CLASSIFICATION OF DISEASES OF THE SKIN

Medical history does not provide many instances in which a father and son wrote and rewrote one book after another on a particular specialty during a span of 60 years. The point of view of the books remained unchangingly that of the practitioner, for, while my father and I held academic positions, our unswerving motivation was to take care of people who came to us for help. In assembling our material, we earnestly squeezed from every scientific contribution that crossed our desks all the information useful to us that we could find in them. The content of many an essay could be put in one or two sentences on a 3x5 file card. Truly there was many a turnip devoid of blood.

The business of bookwriting is arduous and egocentric. When I was a boy, my mother, little sister, and I would keep our home quiet while my father wrote new editions. He wrote some of them in hot summer days before air conditioning was commonplace while seated in a tub of cool water, an ironing board for a desk. He would do a new edition in a few weeks of explosive energy. Then the household would revert to normal, varied from time to time by one of his hunting excursions to Africa, India, Indo-China, or Spitsbergen, which provided museum material for the University of Kansas at Lawrence, the University of Missouri at Columbia, the Kansas City Museum, or our residence. Some of his trophies inspired a prenuptual agreement that my fiancée would not be asked to use tiger skins for rugs or to decorate her walls with rhinoceros faces. Having then much to learn, I got little *quid pro quo*.

When I had completed a bright and shining education, my father employed me in his office. I lived at home, enjoyed free room and board, and was given a Chevrolet automobile and $100 a month. I never had it so good! I married in 1935. My parents approved of their new daughter and gave me $200 a month, but I had to move out.

When I first entered my father's office, freshly trained by Harold N. Cole of Cleveland, Ohio, by Sir Norman Walker and his associates, Cranston Low, Freddie Gardiner, Robert Aitken, and George Hector Percival of the Edinburgh Royal Infirmary (my fellow in training then was Grant Peterkin), and by Col. W. F. Harvey, I.M.S., pathologist of the Royal College of Physicians of

Edinburgh, I sought to acquaint myself with the scientific material my father had accumulated.

"Where are the sections you used in some of your studies?" I asked.

"Over there," he replied, pointing to a pile of small wooden boxes, arranged, if hyperbole may be permitted, like a squirrel's nest. I looked at one, and at others, and found not one label. I chose a slide at random and put it under my father's old Leitz monocular with its rotating circular stage.

"What is this?" I asked. "By golly!" he exclaimed glancing through the eyepiece, "That's old Ben Weber of WaKeeney, Kansas. He had the best damned dogs I ever shot over!"

This unbelievable memory could not be competed with, so I became a labeller. I labelled just about everything I touched from then on.

There were two results. First, our four children, after reading a psychiatry text, labelled me. "Obsessive-compulsive" was their diagnosis. It is true that I straighten tines of restaurant forks but am otherwise socially well adjusted. Secondly, I acquired skills needed for arranging the files of abstracts for the 30,000 or so bibliographic entries in *Diseases of the Skin,* eleventh edition, 1956, as noted in its preface. After its publication a number of friends said to me, "I think I'll write a book someday, Dick. Who did your library work for you?"

Medical writing of this sort requires speed, precision, and pertinacity. When I showed the first copy of the eleventh edition to our family, our youngest daughter said, "Daddy, you've been writing that book all my life." In telling this story, I am in truth making an apology to the child—now a woman with children of her own. I was aware of her existence during those years, and I did love her as dearly as our two older daughters and our son, who received in their early years rather more of my attention.

When I was my father's employee—happy, busy years they were—new patients came to see him, of course, not me. It was perhaps five years until the public perceived that I was alive. My father would chat with a patient briefly, then buzz for me.

"This is my son," he would say, "and his education is far better than my own" (true, I suppose, and I am most grateful). "Son, take this patient out and cure him." These words of his define the purpose of our professional lives.

In 1931 my father handed me his "Big Red Book," eighth edition, and said, "Son, make a little book out of this, for medical students."

I did so. It was a salutary experience, for I learned how bad a book an amateur can write and, too, how much a big book can be condensed without much damaging its message. Early in 1932, there appeared the first edition of *An Introduction to Dermatology.* I was a very young man and so was inordinately pleased with myself. My father was occupied at that time with his hunting or fishing. I sent copies of the book to a number of his friends and mine, enclosing with each a letter inviting the recipient to tell me what he found wrong so that a subsequent edition might be better. Dr. Joseph Grindon, Sr., of St. Louis, who I learned escaped the Jesuit priesthood narrowly, was amazingly obliging. He sent me, after a time, five typescript pages single-spaced of errata, including the correction of all the Latin that had been mismanaged, not all of which was my fault, for I have always transcribed faithfully, giving credit where credit was due. My thank you letter to Dr. Grindon was humble.

Subsequent editions became more and more to my liking; I have been my severest critic. While I have wished to know what others think, I have never felt an obligation to concur.

The prefaces of the books on diseases of the skin that my father and I published during the sixty year period, 1916 to 1975 inclusive, provide historical vignettes of the course and progress of the specialty.

In the prefaces that authors write (but which are seldom read, they suspect) they exploit their prerogative of defining their viewpoint and purpose and their privilege of pointing to inspirations of their own such as they may have cached amid the treasures borrowed from colleagues, artfully arranged and conscientiously accredited. Here I emphasize our contribution of the etiologic classification of dermatologic diseases, first submitted in the preface of the third edition of our *Introduction* in 1937. Classification continued to be etiologic, within the capabilities of the art, in all subsequent books of ours.

Why this is not merely desirable but in truth necessary if skin diseases are to make sense is explained in prefaces of 1937 and thereafter. Actually, the layman is wise enough to speak etiologically of "sunburn," "mosquito bites," and "poison ivy."

I do not wish to put here an essay on the history of dermatologic classification. It is easy to look up. It was presented with especial historical and literary skill by Cecilia C. Mettler. Her *History of Medicine* was published, after her unexpected death in 1943, by Fred A. Mettler (Philadelphia, Blakeston, 1947). See also William A. Pusey's *History of Dermatology* (Springfield, Ill., Charles C. Thomas, 1933).

Mettler traced the progress of dermatology from the classic period through mediaeval times into the 18th and 19th centuries when, with the evolution of the medical sciences, symptomatic listing gave way to arrangements based on pathology. No possibility of etiologic classification existed until microbiology had been developed. Not long thereafter occupational diseases and rashes due to drugs were recognized. Mettler gave photography due credit for promoting luxuriance of the varieties of dermatoses.

The classification of Hieronymus Mercurialis in his *De Morbis Cutaneis* of 1572 followed that of Cornelius Celsus of fifteen centuries previously, dividing skin diseases into those affecting the body and those affecting the head (see Arch. Dermat. 94: 763-772, Dec. 1966).

The subject of classification was reviewed by Robert Jackson of Ottawa (Canadian Med. Assn. Jour. May 21, 1977, p. 1165 ff). Lawrence Charles Parish, of Philadelphia, placed into my hands a lecture by H. D. Bulkley given in 1842 to the New York College of Physicians and Surgeons (published by William E. Dean of New York). His classification followed closely that of Willan, who, like others, was carried away by the botanists and came up with, for example, "Order V, Pustulae, Genus 3, Ecthyma, Species 3, Luridum"—goodness knows what "luridum" was, but the dictionary indicates "ghastly" or "gaudy." (See biography of Willan by John E. Lanc, Arch. Dermet. & Syph. 13: 737-760, 1926.) Biett, a student of Alibert's but much influenced by Willan, than whom in classification he was somewhat more restrained, listed smallpox, impetigo, and acne in his Order IV, Pustulae.

Such obsolete classifications and nomenclatures that mimic the Linnaean are by now obviously fatuous, "eczema rubrum" and the like. The lumping of all scaly lesions is equally devoid of contemporary depth of comprehension.

Erasmus Wilson, a keen observer and articulate, was caught up in the intellectual eddies of his era and mistook what we call pathology for what he called etiology in his *On Diseases of the Skin* of 1843 and 1847.

I ought in clarity to refrain from quoting classificatory miscegenations of some of my contemporaries, whose tables of contents show their quandary when they sought coherence of arrangement, if they did. Oliver Ormsby in the last edition of his *Diseases of the Skin* (Phila., Lea and Febiger, 1956) used essentially the classification of Hebra of the previous century, which at that time had been done as well as it could be done. Ormsby classified responses of the skin as an organ by histopathological criteria. His table of contents included such major subdivisions as hyperemias, inflammations, hypertrophies, atrophies, the pigmentary, metabolic, and neoplastic disorders, nervous and parasitic diseases, and diseases of the skin appendages including the mucous membranes.

In the formal discussions of such major divisions of a dermatologic text as diseases of the hair, or nails, or mucous membranes, they should be presented in etiologic subdivisions, just as diseases of the skin are presented.

It must be conceded that school teachers have their problems. Using their visual and tactile clues, the elementary and secondary lesions (which are extraordinarily difficult to list exhaustively and to define with precision), they must metaphorically put little fingers patiently on the keyboards. But professionals deserve to be addressed at the professional level.

Pity the patient whose therapeutic morphologist appreciates no distinction between the pustules of boils and those of acne—they do look alike until you look close—and the patient who is treated with compresses for oozy diseases and with salves for what's scaly only because his doctor recalls a "pearl" he saw in an elementary reader.

The orderly array of known varieties of causes is useful as well as instructive. It is a checklist for trying to figure out what is the matter with the patient. One reflects, "Is this trouble due to external influences? Could it have been caused by physical agents, chemical agents, or externally active pathogenic organisms? May it represent internal infection, systemic disease, nutritional or glandular derangement, or toxic substances? Does it signify a defect of the blood or vessels, nervous system, or psyche? Is it a kind of malformation or neoplasm? Can it result from any combination of such causes? Why is this individual's skin vulnerable?" I quote the above from Sutton and Waisman's *Practitioners' Dermatology.*

"Prior to the work of Louis Pasteur (1822-95), infections would not have appeared in such a catalogue. We may be sure that some kinds of causes are unknown to us at present" (this from the Doubleday *Handbook* of 1962).

Continuing the line of thought of Sutton and Waisman 1975, but abbreviating, I quote seriatim what I wish to call general solutions of standard problems of treatment for each etiologic class of diseases.

"If the skin is injured, further injury must be averted, infection prevented, and suffering relieved, allowing time for damaged tissues to undergo the physiologic activities of repair.

"If the skin is immediately endangered by a chemical, this must be flooded off at once and further exposure to it prevented. A corticosteroid drug may be expected to reduce the vigor of an inflammatory reaction. Infection must be prevented and suffering relieved while the tissues heal. Injurious chemicals should be identified so that they can be avoided with assurance.

"If the skin is infected, the objectives are to eliminate injurious microorganisms by mechanical, chemical, or biologic means, to alter the host-parasite equilibrium to the advantage of the one and the detriment of the other, to prevent complications and secondary infections, to relieve suffering while the patient's tissues undergo repair, and to prevent infection of other persons. The best plan of treatment may be contingent upon identifying the invader, but measures judged likely to succeed may be exploited even if the pathogen is not as yet known. . . .

"In the disorders of biochemistry, nutrition, endocrine function, and systemic diseases with cutaneous manifestations, therapy aims at correcting the underlying abnormality. It may suffice to improve the diet by supplementing it with protein, vitamins, or iron and other minerals, but an individual correctly fed may nevertheless fail to absorb or utilize what he swallows. Enteropathy and malabsorption as well as proteinuria may accompany extensive dermatoses. Effective endocrine substances or synthetic analogues will supplement deficiencies, among them thyroid, estrogenic and androgenic hormones, insulin, and corticosteroids.

"When allergic sensitization is the essential problem, identification of the allergen usually makes possible its successful avoidance. Specific hyposensitization is seldom effectual in dealing with such dermatoses . . .

"In abnormalities of the psyche, the dermatologist may be amateur yet not entirely helpless. He recognizes the psychosomatic aspects of many dermatologic problems, some of which represent deep psychologic aberration, requiring the care that psychiatrists are best equipped to offer.

"In abnormalities of structure or growth, the patient with a built-in defect needs instruction in how best to live with it. For hereditary diseases, genetic counseling should be provided. Abnormal growths that are not mere blemishes are to be destroyed, if possible, by means of surgery, radiation, or chemotherapy.

"In disorders known to be of unknown cause, many empirical remedies of estimable merit have evolved from trial and error, such as the antimalarials in lupus erythematosus and the sulfones in dermatitis herpetiformis.

"When the joint effects of several causes exist, complicated dermatoses result that are commoner than those of simple etiology. Devising treatment effective for them is like working a combination lock: all the right things must be done at the right time. Etiologic factors that are often overlooked include inconspicuous infection, nutritional deficiency, fatigue, and the patient's feelings about his life situation, the spouse, the boss, the job, the compensation. The exhausted patient does not do well. Caffeine increases irritability of the whole nervous system, including that of the skin. Patients try to hide their addictions to alcohol, tranquilizers, and other drugs . . .

"In managing the recalcitrant case, one asks, 'What interferes with healing, and what can I do about it?' Taking over a patient who has not done well under another doctor's care, one asks, 'What has been tried that didn't work?' and 'What has been overlooked that I must find?' No matter what is wrong, one strives for an optimum state of health by attacking all significant defects that thorough examination uncovers.

"Any case of chronic dermatitis will almost surely improve, regardless of its obscure or unknown cause, if treatment controls contact irritation, eliminates infection, improves nutrition, corrects endocrine glandular abnormalities, remedies discernible systemic disease, eradicates hidden infection, palliates an atopic background if present, provides for adequate rest and emotional calm, and does no harm."

"We do not know the causes of a great many skin diseases, even in our enlightened twentieth century," a critic will say.

"I have never felt more exact," I reply, "than when I know that I don't know, and admit it." It is ignorance of which the owner is ignorant that possesses grandeur. "Do the best you can with what you've got." The next generation will do better.

In no way but by coherent etiologic thinking can plans of treatment be designed that are based on comprehension of the biological and medical sciences.

Among competent practitioners are individuals who are not enamoured of classifications of any sort. It is difficult to refute the proposition that the ideologic web is man-made. I do not recall the mention of classification in any review of a dermatological text. The matter appears to be of little interest in the twentieth century, but it seems important to me.

Nomenclature would undergo a noteworthy upgrading if etiologic principles were a primary consideration. Look at an ordinary conversation with a patient. Would you tell him that he suffers from creep girdle, or girdle-creep (herpes zoster in Greek—choose the adjective for yourself), or rather that he has a segmental infection of the skin with *Herpesvirus varicellae?* Or that it is the red pelt disease (erysipelas in Greek) rather than streptococcic cellulitis of the skin? Or that it is the ruddy wolf disease (lupus erythematosus, if you like your Latin and Greek mixed), rather than auto-immune disease of a particular kind?

The venerable names are obsolescent, indeed superfluous, because you are obliged to translate them, consciously or subconsciously, into etiologic concepts before you can design a regimen likely to succeed.

To assuage the feelings of those who yearn for standardization of nomenclature, precedents may be adduced indicative of the fact that names have a way of passing into oblivion. Our dermatologic forefathers found meanings, satisfactory to them, in names such as mentagra, porrigo, tetter, St. Anthony's fire, herpes tonsurans maculosus, and a hundred others. To exercise the imagination, when would you say the name "streptococcic cellulitis of the skin" would go out of date? "Ringworm" and "tinea" (from Latin *taenia* for grub worm) ought to go. Sabouraud was not etymologically discriminating when he entitled his treatise, "Les Teignes."

Etiologic classification is historically the scientifically sophisticated culmination of arrangement, which through the ages has ranged from the criterion of mere location, through that of the appearance of visible lesions, and thence to the types of microscopic structure.

Dermatology illuminated by etiologic comprehension, even if this is as yet incomplete, makes sense. Therefore it is easier to master, easier to teach, and easier to use effectually for the benefit of those for whom it cares.

# Medical Books
## TITLE PAGES AND PREFACES

# DISEASES OF THE SKIN

BY

RICHARD L. SUTTON, M.D.

PROFESSOR OF DISEASES OF THE SKIN, UNIVERSITY OF KANSAS SCHOOL OF MEDICINE; FORMER CHAIRMAN OF THE DERMATOLOGICAL SECTION OF THE AMERICAN MEDICAL ASSOCIATION; MEMBER AMERICAN DERMATOLOGICAL ASSOCIATION; ASSISTANT SURGEON, UNITED STATES NAVY, RETIRED; DERMATOLOGIST TO THE CHRISTIAN CHURCH HOSPITAL.

*WITH SIX HUNDRED AND NINETY-THREE ILLUSTRATIONS, AND EIGHT COLORED PLATES.*

ST. LOUIS
C. V. MOSBY COMPANY
1916

# PREFACE.

The present volume is the outgrowth of several years of study along this particular line, and is an attempt to present the entire subject of dermatology in a comprehensive, and, at the same time, concise manner.

A treatise covering so broad a field as that of diseases of the skin cannot well be based entirely on the personal knowledge and observations of any single individual. For this reason I have not hesitated to draw from the publications of other writers, selecting the material which I considered most appropriate. Every effort has been made to properly credit the ideas thus secured, and if any mistakes have been committed I trust they will be forgiven.

The symptomatology, diagnosis, and treatment of the various disorders are presented as clearly and simply as possible, and in the manner that I have found most effective in my college and university work.

Particular emphasis has been placed on pathology and treatment. As one of the pioneers in cutaneous medicine has said, no other organ of the body offers such inducements to the pathologist for study as the skin, and for this reason I have devoted more than the usual amount of space to this particular phase of the subject. The majority of the therapeutic measures recommended are those which I have found useful and practicable in my own private and dispensary practice.

The intention has been to advise rather than confuse the less experienced practitioner. Obsolete methods, and those of questionable value or of theoretical interest only, are discussed briefly and frankly, or omitted altogether.

Owing to the number of references given, it was thought best to dispense with numbered text citations. The appended lists of references will be found to contain practically all of the more important contributions to our knowledge of the various subjects, and have been carefully checked over by Mrs. Rose Hibbard, and her assistant, Miss Elizabeth Cogswell, of the Kansas City Medical Library Club. I believe them to be accurate.

I am under obligation to Dr. George H. Simmons, Editor of the *Journal of the American Medical Association,* for permission to use several articles which were previously published in the Journal. I am also deeply indebted to numerous colleagues and friends in various parts of the world for placing at my disposal their collections of photographs from which I have drawn freely.

While the greater amount of space has been devoted to the illustration of examples of the commoner disorders, such as eczema and syphilis, the rarer dermatoses have not been neglected, as examination will show. Several of these, such as uta, or espundia, cutaneous thrush, foot-and-mouth disease, and trichinosis, have never before been pictorially represented in any book, and I trust will prove of value from a diagnostic point of view.

RICHARD L. SUTTON.

Kansas City, Mo.

# DISEASES OF THE SKIN

BY

RICHARD L. SUTTON, M.D.

PROFESSOR OF DISEASES OF THE SKIN, UNIVERSITY OF KANSAS SCHOOL OF MEDICINE; FORMER CHAIRMAN OF THE DERMATOLOGICAL SECTION OF THE AMERICAN MEDICAL ASSOCIATION; MEMBER AMERICAN DERMATOLOGICAL ASSOCIATION; ASSISTANT SURGEON, UNITED STATES NAVY, RETIRED; DERMATOLOGIST TO THE CHRISTIAN CHURCH HOSPITAL.

*WITH EIGHT HUNDRED AND THIRTY-THREE ILLUSTRATIONS, AND EIGHT COLORED PLATES.*

SECOND EDITION, REVISED AND ENLARGED.

ST. LOUIS
C. V. MOSBY COMPANY
1917

# PREFACE TO SECOND EDITION.

The demand for a second edition at this time has given me opportunity to supply supplemental matter in a few instances, as well as to cover the important literature for the entire year of 1916, and eliminate a number of typographic and other minor errors.

Among new topics considered are Gangrenous Balanitis, Atrophy of the Mucous Membranes of the Tongue and Mouth, and Atrophy of the Fatty Layer of the Skin. The article on Perlèche has been re-written, and that portion of the one on pediculosis which deals with treatment, considerably amplified.

Through the liberality of my publishers, one hundred and forty new illustrations have been added.

I am deeply grateful to my friends and colleagues for the kind and generous reception accorded the first edition, and I sincerely hope that the present one will be found to fill a need in modern dermatologic literature.

RICHARD L. SUTTON.

# DISEASES OF THE SKIN

BY

RICHARD L. SUTTON, M.D.

PROFESSOR OF DISEASES OF THE SKIN, UNIVERSITY OF KANSAS SCHOOL OF MEDICINE; FORMER CHAIRMAN OF THE DERMATOLOGICAL SECTION OF THE AMERICAN MEDICAL ASSOCIATION; ASSISTANT SURGEON, UNITED STATES NAVY, RETIRED; DERMATOLOGIST TO THE CHRISTIAN CHURCH HOSPITAL.

*WITH NINE HUNDRED TEN ILLUSTRATIONS, AND ELEVEN COLORED PLATES.*

THIRD EDITION, REVISED AND ENLARGED.

ST. LOUIS
C. V. MOSBY COMPANY
1919

# PREFACE TO THE THIRD EDITION.

In this edition an effort has been made to cover all of the important dermatological literature up to the beginning of the present year. While the war has had a deterrent effect upon the study of cutaneous medicine in general, it has added to our knowledge of the successful management of a few disorders, notably those due to animal parasites; and has developed a few new affections, such as occupation and traumatic dermatoses due to tetryl, dichlorethylsulphide and similar chemical irritants, and inflammatory and trophic disturbances resulting from long continued exposure to adverse atmospheric conditions.

The gravity of syphilis as a social disease is becoming more evident each year—a fact to which attention has been called by the splendid contributions of William Allen Pusey, John H. Stokes, Loyd Thompson, H. H. Hazen, and other authorities—and for this reason the malady has been accorded an even greater amount of space than in previous editions.

The important part played by focal infections of the teeth, tonsils, prostate, and other organs, in the causation of disorders of the skin, is at last becoming generally recognized; and I have endeavored to emphasize such a relationship in those conditions where it is known to exist.

Among the more recently discovered diseases of the skin, Erythema Figuratum Perstans, Necrobacillosis of the Skin, Folliculitis Ulerythematosa Reticulata, Barcoo Rot, Chondro-dermatitis Nodularis Chronica Helicis, and Retention Cysts of the Mucous Membrane of the Lip are described.

I am indebted to many colleagues for valued suggestions and advice, and particularly to my friend, Dr. Charles J. White, of Boston, whose encouragement and example have been constant sources of inspiration during my entire dermatological career.

Through the generosity of the publishers I have been enabled to add eighty new illustrations. The four hundred additional references to the literature have been carefully checked by Mrs. Rosa Hibbard, of the Kansas City Medical Library Club, and I believe will be found of value to research students and others who may desire to investigate exhaustively any particular subject.

RICHARD L. SUTTON.

# DISEASES OF THE SKIN

BY

RICHARD L. SUTTON, M.D.

PROFESSOR OF DISEASES OF THE SKIN, UNIVERSITY OF KANSAS SCHOOL OF MEDICINE; FORMER CHAIRMAN OF THE DERMATOLOGICAL SECTION OF THE AMERICAN MEDICAL ASSOCIATION; ASSISTANT SURGEON, UNITED STATES NAVY, RETIRED; DERMATOLOGIST TO THE CHRISTIAN CHURCH HOSPITAL.

*WITH NINE HUNDRED SIXTY-NINE ILLUSTRATIONS, AND ELEVEN COLORED PLATES*

FOURTH EDITION, REVISED AND ENLARGED

ST. LOUIS
C. V. MOSBY COMPANY
1921

18

# PREFACE TO THE FOURTH EDITION.

While no startling discoveries in medicine have been made during the past two years, a survey of the literature shows that our knowledge of dermatology has steadily and consistently advanced along many lines.

The clinical and serological study of syphilis continues to hold the attention of a large and able body of investigators, and the general public is at last beginning to appreciate the widespread prevalence and disastrous consequences of this malady.

The researches of Ormsby and Mitchell, Charles J. White, Wende and Wilkinson, and others, on epidermophyton infection and its etiologic relationship to certain chronic, inflammatory disorders of the skin, have served to call attention to an important field which has hitherto been sadly neglected in this country.

Descriptions of nocardiosis, Vincent's disease, dermatitis dysmenorrheica, amebiasis cutis, and neurotic excoriations of the skin will be found under new headings.

Owing to the large amount of valuable new material which must be considered, it has been necessary to conserve space in every possible manner. For this reason, some of the domestic literature which is easy of access has not received the full attention that its quality deserves, while certain foreign contributions, far less important, have been abstracted more liberally because of their inaccessibility to the average reader.

Through the generosity of the publishers, and the courtesy of various colleagues, I have been enabled to add a number of new illustrations. The six hundred forty additional references have been carefully checked by Mrs. Rosa Hibbard, of the Kansas City Medical Library Club, and I trust will be of value to students and others who may desire to exhaustively investigate any particular subject.

RICHARD L. SUTTON.

# DISEASES OF THE SKIN

BY
RICHARD L. SUTTON, M.D., LL.D.,

PROFESSOR OF DISEASES OF THE SKIN, UNIVERSITY OF KANSAS SCHOOL OF MEDICINE; FORMER CHAIRMAN OF THE DERMATOLOGICAL SECTION OF THE AMERICAN MEDICAL ASSOCIATION; ASSISTANT SURGEON, UNITED STATES NAVY, RETIRED; DERMATOLOGIST TO THE CHRISTIAN CHURCH HOSPITAL.

*WITH ONE THOUSAND SIXTY-NINE ILLUSTRATIONS, AND ELEVEN COLORED PLATES*

FIFTH EDITION, REVISED AND ENLARGED

C. V. MOSBY COMPANY
ST. LOUIS
1923

## PREFACE TO THE FIFTH EDITION.

To one who has had a watchful finger on the pulse of dermatological literature for a decade and a half, the output for the past two years is as promising as it has been prolific.

The most pleasing feature of all has been the large percentage of contributions emanating from the younger generation of dermatologists, particularly here in America.

The fields that have been investigated since the publication of the fourth edition have been both varied and extensive. Syphilis continues to hold the attention of a large and able body of workers, so large in fact that the resulting literature is rapidly becoming too bulky for exhaustive consideration in any one volume treatise on dermatology. The importance of ringworm as a causative factor in many hitherto obscure cutaneous disorders is becoming generally recognized.

Descriptions of alastrim, itchy points, erosio interdigitalis blastomycetica, poikiloderma atrophicans vasculare, melanotic whitlow, multiple benign tumor-like new growths of the skin, Rocky Mountain fever, the pink disease, perifolliculitis capitis abscedens et suffodens, wit-kop, ochronosis, carotinoid pigmentation of the skin, and hypodermiasis will be found under new headings.

Through the courtesy and generosity of the publishers, about one hundred new illustrations have been added. A few of these have been used to replace older, and less characteristic, photographs. I am indebted to my son, Richard L. Sutton, Jr., for many of the photomicrographs. Without his enthusiastic aid and cooperation, they never would have been made. The six hundred new literary references have been carefully selected from a list of several thousand, and I trust will be of value to research students and others who may wish to exhaustively investigate any particular subject.

RICHARD L. SUTTON.

KANSAS CITY, 1923.

# DISEASES OF THE SKIN

BY

RICHARD L. SUTTON, M.D., LL.D., F.R.S.(EDIN.),

PROFESSOR OF DISEASES OF THE SKIN, UNIVERSITY OF KANSAS SCHOOL OF MEDICINE; ASSISTANT SURGEON, UNITED STATES NAVY, RETIRED; MEMBER OF THE AMERICAN DERMATOLOGICAL ASSOCIATION; DERMATOLOGIST TO THE ATCHISON, TOPEKA AND SANTA FE HOSPITAL ASSOCIATION; DERMATOLOGIST TO THE CHRISTIAN CHURCH HOSPITAL.

*WITH 1147 ILLUSTRATIONS, AND 11 COLORED PLATES*

SIXTH EDITION

REVISED AND ENLARGED

ST. LOUIS

THE C. V. MOSBY COMPANY

1926

22

## PREFACE TO THE SIXTH EDITION.

More than two years have elapsed since the publication of the fifth edition, and the quality and the amount of new material that has accumulated in the interval speak well for the ability and industry of the men who are interested in this important branch of medicine.

With the adoption of modern methods of investigation, our views on many of the subjects have considerably altered, and for this reason I have endeavored to get rid of much of the old matter that has become obsolete.

Additional light is constantly being thrown on a number of cutaneous disorders, and while our therapeutic advances have not kept pace with the information gained along other lines, we at least are in position to combat the various mycotic disorders far more intelligently, if not more successfully, than we were half a decade ago.

The literature dealing with syphilis in its various phases and manifestations has become so voluminous that only an encyclopedia especially devoted to the subject could begin to do it justice, consequently I have refrained from discussing it in minute detail, and confined myself wholly to a practical consideration of the diagnosis, and modern methods of treatment..

A few of the rarer or more recently discovered dermatoses, as Fox-Fordyce disease, mycotic paronychia (Kingery-Thienes), congenital ectodermal aplasia, cheilitis actinica chronica (Ayres), ulcus vulvae acutum, glossitis rhombica mediana, achromia parasitica, and the dermatologic aspect of rat-bite fever are included for the first time.

Through the courtesy and generosity of the publishers, a number of new photographs and photomicrographs have been added. For practically all of the latter, I am indebted to my son, Richard L. Sutton, Jr.

About eight hundred new literary references have been appended; and as these have been carefully selected from a very long list, and carefully checked, I trust they will prove of value to research students and others who may wish to exhaustively investigate any particular subject.

RICHARD L. SUTTON.

KANSAS CITY, 1926.

# DISEASES OF THE SKIN

BY

RICHARD L. SUTTON, M.D., Sc.D., LL.D., F.R.S. (EDIN.),

Professor of Diseases of the Skin, University of Kansas School of Medicine; Assistant Surgeon, United States Navy, Retired; Member of the American Dermatological Association; Dermatologist to The Santa Fe Hospital Association; Dermatologist to the Bell Memorial Hospital, the Swofford Home for Children, the Nettleton and Armour Homes for the Aged, and Visiting Dermatologist to the Kansas City General Hospital.

*WITH 1237 ILLUSTRATIONS, AND 11 COLORED PLATES*

SEVENTH EDITION

REVISED AND ENLARGED

ST. LOUIS

THE C. V. MOSBY COMPANY

1928

24

# PREFACE TO THE SEVENTH EDITION

At the time of the publication of the sixth edition, it was thought that a new impression once in every three years would be sufficient to take care of all future needs, but the continued indulgent reception accorded the work, together with the accumulation of a large amount of new and valuable material, has rendered this plan impracticable. Several recently discovered diseases have been introduced, the descriptions of some of the older ones rewritten, and the importance of others, such as certain of the occupational dermatoses, and those related to allergy, emphasized.

An attempt has been made to discuss intelligently the latest developments in cutaneous therapy, and to recommend those agents known to be reliable, and practicable. Much that is of theoretical interest only has been left out. A textbook is no place for the discussion of experimental medicine. It is difficult enough for the harassed medical student to remember the useful things. He should not be asked to burden his mind with a horde of unproved theories, many of which ultimately will be found worthless, if not actually dangerous.

Owing to the increase in size of each new edition, I have endeavored to get rid of all obsolete matter, and to condense the new material as much as is consistent with clarity. In order to further economize space, a considerable number of valuable references have had to be confined wholly to footnotes, otherwise the volume would soon become so bulky and unwieldy as to seriously impair its usefulness.

I am grateful to many colleagues for valuable suggestions and advice, and particularly to Dr. George Miller MacKee, Dr. Howard Fox, and Dr. Samuel Sweitzer, for their generosity regarding illustrations. Dr. Frederick D. Weidman has been so kind as to permit the use of a large and previously unpublished collection of interesting photomicrographs, and Dr. Stuart Way, and my son, Richard L. Sutton, Jr., also have contributed new ones. The references have been carefully checked, and will, I trust, prove of value to the research worker as well as to the undergraduate student.

RICHARD L. SUTTON.

KANSAS CITY, MISSOURI.

# DISEASES OF THE SKIN

BY

RICHARD L. SUTTON, M.D., Sc.D., LL.D., F.R.S. (EDIN.)

Professor of Diseases of the Skin, University of Kansas School of Medicine; Assistant Surgeon, United States Navy, Retired; Member of the American Dermatological Association; Dermatologist to The Santa Fe Hospital Association; Dermatologist to the Bell Memorial Hospital, the Spofford Home for Children, the Nettleton and Armour Homes for the Aged, and Visiting Dermatologist to the Kansas City General Hospital

*WITH 1290 ILLUSTRATIONS, AND 11 COLORED PLATES*

EIGHTH EDITION

REVISED AND ENLARGED

ST. LOUIS

THE C. V. MOSBY COMPANY

1931

# PREFACE TO THE EIGHTH EDITION.

The author of a textbook on so young and vigorous a specialty as dermatology faces a grave responsibility. The volume must serve as a reference work as well as a clinical and therapeutic guide to both the medical student and the active practitioner of medicine. To be of value, it should be practical, as well as concise. Controversy must be avoided, needless detail omitted, and questions which are of theoretical importance only, ignored.

Modern dermatological literature appears to grow by leaps and bounds. An exhaustive review of the original contributions published during a single year would fill a medium sized volume. On the other hand, it is essential that each new edition contain an easily accessible and complete record of all the authoritative reports that have appeared in the interval. This I have endeavored to do, to the best of my ability, but even the most skilled of phraseological artists will experience difficulty in condensing and crystallizing the wisdom of a three thousand word masterpiece into the space of one or two brief sentences, and I must acknowledge that I am no literary Cellini. Scanning the completed task, no one realizes better than I how incompletely it fulfills the ideal.

Through the courtesy and ingenuity of my publishers, the present edition has been considerably lessened in both size and weight, a result of the rearrangement of the illustrations, and the use of a somewhat lighter and finer grade of paper. I trust that this change will meet with the approval of the reader.

Owing to the fact that the roentgen ray and similar powerful agents can safely be employed only by an operator who has had a certain amount of practical training, I have thought it unwise to devote a large amount of space simply to didactic description.

I am indebted to Drs. Kessler and Kessler, Stuart C. Way, Howard Fox, Everett S. Lain, Hamilton Montgomery, Samuel E. Sweitzer and others of my friends for much new illustrative material, and, as in previous editions, to my son, Dr. Richard L. Sutton, Jr., for helpful suggestions and advice.

R. L. S.

Kansas City, Missouri.

# AN INTRODUCTION
TO
# DERMATOLOGY

BY

RICHARD L. SUTTON
M.D., Sc.D., LL.D., F.R.S. (EDIN.)

PROFESSOR OF DISEASES OF THE SKIN, UNIVERSITY OF KANSAS
SCHOOL OF MEDICINE

AND

RICHARD L. SUTTON, JR., A.M., M.D.

VISITING DERMATOLOGIST TO THE KANSAS CITY GENERAL HOSPITAL

*WITH 183 ILLUSTRATIONS*

ST. LOUIS
THE C. V. MOSBY COMPANY
**1932**

# PREFACE

This book is intended primarily for students. After having taught dermatology for a fifth of a century, I am convinced that it is not wise to ask a student to plunge himself into the intricacies of a thousand or twelve hundred page textbook, and to pick out from this volume the fundamentals of dermatology. On the other hand, my experience has taught me that it is much better for the writer of a textbook to sift, to cull, to condense, and then to offer the essentials upon which a sound knowledge of dermatology can be built. After this foundation has been laid, then I would recommend a book which is mainly clinical, a book replete with illustrations that make a differential diagnosis and a rational plan of treatment possible.

In the preparation of this volume, which is based on the eighth edition of my textbook *Diseases of the Skin,* I have depended almost entirely upon my son and associate, Dr. Richard L. Sutton, Jr., a recent graduate in medicine, who for several years has been deeply interested in dermatology.

In my opinion, the most instructive medical books are those which have been written by men who are still able to recognize and appreciate the viewpoint of both the student and the confirmed specialist. A volume composed by a young and unsophisticated man may be more readily understood by the student, but generally it is lacking in those practical elements which only time and actual experience can supply. On the other hand, a physician who in his later years writes a book is very liable to take too much for granted, and to feel that his reader already is conversant with matter which to him appears mere kindergarten material but which to the unfortunate average student is Greek.

For this reason, we have endeavored to combine judiciously the old and the new, retaining the original lattice work of fundamental facts which contributed so much to the value and popularity of the parent volume, and omitting much descriptive and statistical matter which is of interest to only the research worker and the specialist.

I trust the resulting manual is one that will meet with the approval not only of the student body, but of practitioners and teachers as well.

RICHARD L. SUTTON.

KANSAS CITY, MISSOURI.

# AN INTRODUCTION
## TO
# DERMATOLOGY

BY

RICHARD L. SUTTON
M.D., Sc.D., LL.D., F.R.S. (EDIN.)

PROFESSOR OF DISEASES OF THE SKIN, UNIVERSITY OF KANSAS
SCHOOL OF MEDICINE

AND

RICHARD L. SUTTON, JR.
A.M., M.D., L.R.C.P. (EDIN.)

ASSISTANT IN DERMATOLOGY, UNIVERSITY OF KANSAS SCHOOL OF MEDICINE

*WITH 190 ILLUSTRATIONS*

SECOND EDITION

ST. LOUIS
THE C. V. MOSBY COMPANY
1933

## PREFACE TO SECOND EDITION

The kind reception accorded the first edition of this book is deeply appreciated by the authors. While it was thought that the volume would fill a distinct need, the enthusiastic welcome which it has received from not only the student and the teacher, but the general medical man as well, has been both surprising and gratifying.

Judging from numerous comments, a large and comprehensive volume for this purpose is not desired. Therefore we shall continue to confine the size of future editions to about that of the first one. In order to do this descriptions of the rarer dermatoses must be condensed, or eliminated altogether, and the illustrations restricted mainly to those which portray only the commoner diseases of the skin.

While some new material has been added, particularly along the line of therapy, care has been taken to omit matter which is of theoretical interest only. The main value of a book of this sort must lie in its conciseness and practicability.

In the present volume, as in the earlier one, I have depended wholly upon the services of my son, Dr. Richard L. Sutton, Jr. My part in the production has been solely that of consultant.

I sincerely trust that the volume will continue to merit the confidence and approbation of our friends and colleagues.

R. L. SUTTON

# DISEASES OF THE SKIN

BY

RICHARD L. SUTTON
M.D., Sc.D., LL.D., F.R.S. (EDIN.)
PROFESSOR OF DERMATOLOGY, UNIVERSITY OF KANSAS, SCHOOL OF MEDICINE

AND

RICHARD L. SUTTON, JR.
A.M., M.D., L.R.C.P. (EDIN.)
ASSISTANT IN DERMATOLOGY, UNIVERSITY OF KANSAS, SCHOOL OF MEDICINE

*WITH 1,310 ILLUSTRATIONS, AND 11 COLORED PLATES*

NINTH EDITION
REVISED AND ENLARGED

ST. LOUIS
THE C. V. MOSBY COMPANY
1935

## PREFACE TO THE NINTH EDITION.

Twenty years ago, when I began collecting material for the first edition of this work, little did I suspect that it would ever grow into the present ponderous volume. Had I done so, it is very probable that I should have tried to content myself with labors that demanded far less time and effort.

A book of this sort is like a child; the author, an anxious and doting parent.

For many years, my son, Richard L. Sutton, Jr., has aided me in the compilation of the various editions, and for that reason I have now adopted him as a permanent literary associate.

In the present volume, he is responsible for the descriptions of those diseases and conditions which are included for the first time (pyodermia gangraenosum, pili torti, telangiectasia macularis eruptiva perstans, cutis rhomboidalis nuchae, cephalosporiosis, pseudoatrophoderma colli, hidrosadenitis axillaris, necrobiosis lipoidica diabeticorum, anaphylactic gangrene, granuloma fissuratum, lingual tonsillitis, psoriatic exfoliative dermatitis, erythema annulare centrifugum, scleredema adultorum, dermatomyositis, calcification in the skin, hemolytic streptococcic gangrene, congenital skin defects of the newborn, calcifying epithelioma, nodular subepidermal fibroses, discrete keratodermia of the hands, ganglioneuroma, amyloidosis of the skin, juvenile elastoma, erythroplasia of Queyrat, brucella dermatitis, traumatic epithelial cysts of the skin, and acquired progressive kinking of the scalp), and the revision of coccidioidal granuloma, tularemia, and the treatment of syphilis, as well as for the new photographs and photomicrographs.

I have supplied the new references, and supervised the arrangement of the material. Every effort has been made to bring the book completely up to date, and to give credit where credit is due. If there are any errors or omissions, I trust they will be forgiven.

We are under obligation to many of our colleagues for new ideas and suggestions, and we wish especially to acknowledge our great indebtedness to the *Archives of Dermatology and Syphilology,* and to its distinguished Editor in Chief, Dr. William Allen Pusey. Without the aid of this admirable publication, I doubt if the book would ever have reached a sixth edition, let alone a ninth. Drs. Charles J. White, Joseph

Grindon, Harold N. Cole, Samuel E. Sweitzer, Erwin P. Zeisler, A. Benson Cannon and others have donated valuable literary and illustrative material.

Needless to say, we are grateful to a host of friends for their indulgence and support.

I can only hope that our efforts will continue to merit their confidence and approval.

R. L. S.

Kansas City, Missouri.

# AN INTRODUCTION
## TO
# DERMATOLOGY


BY

RICHARD L. SUTTON
M.D., Sc.D., LL.D., F.R.S. (EDIN.)

PROFESSOR OF DERMATOLOGY, UNIVERSITY OF KANSAS
SCHOOL OF MEDICINE

AND

RICHARD L. SUTTON, JR.
A.M., M.D., L.R.C.P. (EDIN.)

INSTRUCTOR IN DERMATOLOGY, UNIVERSITY OF KANSAS SCHOOL OF MEDICINE


THIRD EDITION


ST. LOUIS
THE C. V. MOSBY COMPANY
1937

# PREFACE TO THE THIRD EDITION

Of all the medical specialties, few have made greater progress in recent years than dermatology. For this reason, a vast amount of new material has accumulated since the publication of the second edition in 1933. As a result, the volume had to be completely rewritten, and changes will be found on almost every page.

A serious attempt at reclassification has been made, as much as possible on the basis of etiology. Several members of the old "inflammation" group have been placed in more appropriate sections, and a few of the hypertrophies have joined the so-called "bacterial" group, while others, such as myxedema, have been included under metabolic disorders.

The parasitic affections have been subdivided into new chapters, and the entire subject generally renovated and brought up to date.

Forty-five new illustrations have been added. Much new information regarding therapy has been introduced.

Descriptions of a number of new diseases are included for the first time: erythema annulare centrifugum, pyoderma gangrenosum, pigmented purpuric lichenoid dermatitis, dermatomyositis, scleredema adultorum, poikiloderma of Civatte, congenital skin defects of the newborn, Mongolian spots, nevoxanthoendothelioma, necrobiosis lipoidica diabeticorum, Addison's disease, pituitary basophilism, calcification in the skin, avitaminosis, cutis rhomboidalis nuchae, amyloidosis cutis, circumscribed myxedema, hemochromatosis, nodular subepidermal fibroses, subcutaneous fat necrosis, glomus tumors, neurilemoma, mixed tumors of the palate, congenital dermal sinuses (including congenital auricular fistulae and pilonidal cysts), calcifying epithelioma, Kaposi's varicelliform eruption, hemolytic streptococcal gangrene, rat mite dermatitis, tick-bite fever, onchocerciasis, bites (fly, mosquito, assassin bug, myriapod, spider), grasshopper dermatitis, blister beetles, onion mite dermatitis, lingual tonsillitis.

The section on syphilis has been enlarged, the important findings of the Cooperative Clinical Group have been discussed, and modern methods of treatment stressed, with particular reference to the value of bismuth.

Atopic eczema, and the relationship of lichen simplex, eczema, and dermatitis venenata are considered in detail; the treatment of infantile eczema has been enlarged and simplified, and the section on animal parasitic diseases has been completely revised. The section on cancer of the skin has been enriched by many new photographs and photomicrographs, together with numerous recent references on diagnosis and treatment.

As in previous editions, I have depended entirely upon my son, Dr. Richard L. Sutton, Jr., in the preparation of this work. My part in the production has been that of consultant and counselor.

We are grateful to our friends and colleagues for their continued confidence and support, and we trust that the present volume will find an even wider field of usefulness.

R. L. Sutton.

# DISEASES OF THE SKIN

BY

RICHARD L. SUTTON

M.D., Sc.D., LL.D., F.R.S. (Edin.)

PROFESSOR OF DERMATOLOGY, UNIVERSITY OF KANSAS, SCHOOL OF MEDICINE

AND

RICHARD L. SUTTON, JR.

A.M., M.D., L.R.C.P. (Edin.)

ASSOCIATE IN DERMATOLOGY, UNIVERSITY OF KANSAS, SCHOOL OF MEDICINE

*WITH 1452 TEXT ILLUSTRATIONS*
*AND 21 COLOR PLATES*

TENTH EDITION

REVISED, ENLARGED AND RESET

ST. LOUIS

THE C. V. MOSBY COMPANY

1939

# PREFACE TO THE TENTH EDITION

Few branches of medicine have made such progress in the past four years as has dermatology. Without losing recognition of this field of practice as a specialty, we believe that the time has come to tie descriptions and concepts of disorders of the skin with general medicine and biology. Here we have attempted to do this. The point of view is taken that the processes of pathology are in general inevitable responses under the circumstances; a furuncle is the normal bodily reaction to virulent staphylococci in a hair follicle. Diseases are three-dimensional moving pictures. Skin diseases are visible tissular activities.

In view of the favorable reception accorded the etiologic classification in the 1937 edition of our *Introduction to Dermatology*, and the tendency nowadays to inquire "What is going on?" rather than "What name is applicable to this manifestation?" the material has been arranged in a fashion radically different from that in the ninth edition.

Descriptions of all significant entities, syndromes, and concepts, and of many exotic, unusual, and even exceptional dermatoses have been incorporated. Emphasis is laid, however, on the purpose of practical medicine, which is to cure the ordinary patient of his ordinary complaints by scientific or by pragmatic means. While the chapters on parasitic dermatoses, plant and animal, have been expanded to meet exacting requirements, the recognition, comprehension, and management of tinea, moniliasis, dermatophytids, scabies, and pediculosis have been clarified, we hope, rather than obscured.

There have been added ten color plates and some three hundred forty new illustrations, many of the new cuts replacing those impaired by wear and tear in previous editions. By condensation of type and efficient use of enlarged page space, a 100 per cent increment in number of words and at least seven thousand bibliographic entries have been added to the rewritten material of the ninth edition.

Attention should be given to the bibliography, in which many comments are included in small type which otherwise would have to have been omitted; these the special student will find of interest.

The comprehensive index is indispensable for cross references.

We have not hesitated to give our opinions, interpretations, and ideas, particularly regarding treatment. In some instances these are original, as in the treatment of acne vulgaris, calcinosis universalis, urticaria pigmentosa, and pityriasis rosea; in the etiology of infantile mycotic eczema as sometimes a birth canal infection; and in the description of keratoses, leucoplakia, and early carcinomas. Other original contributions include squamous-cell keratosis, congenital fistulas of the labial commissures, the most extensive recorded case of naevus follicularis keratosis.

A brief descriptive style has been adhered to, for a treatise of one volume, unlike a system, is limited in its allowance of space.

Dr. Charles R. Rein contributed the section on serologic diagnosis of syphilis, giving the reagents used and the methods of their use. This material is included for the ready access of the inquisitive physician rather than primarily for the laboratory technician, although it is complete.

Dr. George M. Lewis and Dr. Mary Hopper, of the New York Skin and Cancer Unit, contributed statements of the cultural characteristics and identifying features of common pathogenic fungi, photographs of giant colonies, and photomicrographs of fungi. We believe that the identification of particular fungous diseases will eventually supplant the less modern diagnostication of tinea.

Dr. Herman E. Hasseltine, Medical Officer in Charge, U. S. Marine Hospital, Carville, Louisiana (the National Leper Home), and his associate, Dr. Frederick A. Johansen, reviewed the manuscript on leprosy at our request and gave us many valuable suggestions.

Col. W. F. Harvey, of the Royal College of Physicians of Edinburgh, by his stimulating interest in tumors and through the facilities of the Laboratory, has enabled us to utilize histologic preparations of whole tumors, exceptional in quality and variety. All new, original photomicrographs have been made from these slides, for which we furnished tissue, notably those depicting the histogenesis of carcinoma.

We have largely followed Dr. E. Brumpt's *Précis de Parasitologie* in our presentation of animal and plant parasitism of the skin. Dr. H. H. Lane, zoologist, of the University of Kansas, checked with us the nomenclature of Chapter XX; but we are responsible for errors which may remain.

Dr. Howard Fox exchanged with us instructive correspondence regarding subcutaneous fat necrosis of the newborn, pinta, leishmaniasis, and other matters. Dr. Harold N. Cole, as in previous editions, has been an invaluable friend and adviser. We have profited by Dr. Earl Osborne's suggestions regarding eczema and allied disorders, and by his constructive criticism of our previous manner of presentation of this material. Dr. Lee McCarthy has generously allowed the use of many valuable plates from his *Histopathology of Skin Diseases.* Dr. Henry H. Hazen permitted us to select a number of photomicrographs of syphilis from his splendid collection. Dr. Louis V. Hayes liberally gave us several illustrations from his *Clinical Diagnosis of Diseases of the Mouth.* Dr. R. B. H. Gradwohl kindly contributed several photomicrographs of parasites. Dr. Jonathan C. Meakins let us use several illustrations from his *Practice of Medicine.* The *Year Book of Dermatology and Syphilology,* edited by Dr. Fred Wise and Dr. Marion B. Sulzberger, has been a welcome labor-saving device.

We are indebted to many persons and to several journals for illustrative material. In each case, acknowledgment has been incorporated within the legend.

The preparation of this revision would have been impossible without the skilled assistance of librarians; in this we have been fortunate. Our indebtedness is gratefully acknowledged to Miss Eleanor Chase, of the Jackson County Medical Society, Miss Opal Woodruff, of the University of Kansas, School of Medicine, and her associates, Miss Dorothy Holt and Mrs. Beulah Nash, and to the Jackson County Medical Society and the University of Kansas.

The C. V. Mosby Company, in resetting the book, in managing the work of bookmaking, and in allowing complete freedom in the addition of illustrations and textual matter, has most cooperatively put its facilities at our command.

We are grateful to our friends and colleagues for their confidence and support, and we trust that the tenth edition will find a wide field of usefulness.

R. L. Sutton
R. L. Sutton, Jr.

# AN INTRODUCTION
# TO
# DERMATOLOGY


BY

RICHARD L. SUTTON
M.D., Sc.D., LL.D., F.R.S. (Edin.)
Emeritus Professor of Dermatology, University of Kansas
School of Medicine

AND

RICHARD L. SUTTON, JR.
A.M., M.D., L.R.C.P. (Edin.)
Assistant Professor of Dermatology, University of Kansas
School of Medicine


*With 723 Illustrations*

Fourth Edition


ST. LOUIS
THE C. V. MOSBY COMPANY
1941

# PREFACE TO THE FOURTH EDITION

This book, intended for students, collegiate and postgraduate, contains a review of dermatology sufficient to outline the scope of the specialty beyond provincial boundaries. It contains considerably more than a student may encompass, but he can always read less of it. If he needs more, the bibliography, an innovation in this edition, is selected to accommodate his desires or assignments.

This fourth edition has been condensed from the tenth edition of our *Diseases of the Skin,* as the first edition of the *Introduction* was condensed from the eighth edition of the comprehensive volume. Modifications have been made, taking into account medical literature which has appeared since the middle of 1939.

Illustration has received our especial effort. Intimate incorporation of figures within text has been sought by including author and journal references in titles in many instances, affording inspiration, we hope, for the reader to examine articles in which figures originally appeared.

The number of illustrations has been more than trebled.

The type has been reset.

The bibliography has been selected with a view to utility. Leading articles of recent date, especially those which themselves incorporate reviews of literature, have been chosen. Most references are to articles in the English language, and journals of wide circulation have been given preference. In view of the availability of libraries and indexes to medical literature in all medical schools, not every contribution to which we have attached the author's name is given actual bibliographic reference, through consideration of the space requirement of extensive lists.

We acknowledge gratefully our indebtedness to many who have kindly permitted our use of their scientific contributions and photographs. Effort has been made to accredit them accurately.

Dr. Hermann Pinkus supplied us with a magnificent collection of photomicrographs of normal adult and embryonic cutaneous tissues from various regions, prepared with various stains. This collection, graciously made at our request, is so extensive that only a part is represented by those we selected for inclusion here. It is our belief that pictures of tissues surpass diagrams and drawings in teaching value.

Dr. Harold N. Cole, Dr. George Miller MacKee, Dr. Howard Fox, Dr. D. E. H. Cleveland, Dr. George M. Lewis, Dr. Mary Hopper, and Dr. F. Ronchese are among those who have responded generously to our requests for material. Dr. Charles Rein has provided descriptions of several serologic tests for syphilis; these are included for the convenience of inquisitive medical persons rather than for the use of laboratory technicians, although they are complete.

PREFACE

Patient and expert aid in preparing the bibliography was given by Miss Eleanor Chase, Librarian of the Jackson County Medical Society Library, by Miss Opal Woodruff, Librarian of the University of Kansas Medical School, and by Miss Dorothea Mattics, our secretary. The C. V. Mosby Company have made the task a cooperative and pleasant one.

R. L. SUTTON, SR.
R. L. SUTTON, JR.

# SYNOPSIS OF DISEASES OF THE SKIN

BY

RICHARD L. SUTTON, M.D.

Emeritus Professor of Dermatology, University of Kansas Medical School

AND

RICHARD L. SUTTON, JR., M.D.

Assistant Professor of Dermatology, University of Kansas Medical School

*WITH 413 ILLUSTRATIONS*

ST. LOUIS

THE C. V. MOSBY COMPANY

1942

# PREFACE

This book is intended to present in compact form a general view of diseases of the skin. We have consolidated and retained essentials and have sought to use the space at our disposal to the greatest possible advantage. Simplicity, practicality, and condensation are the aims, dwelling longest on the elementary and the commonplace, least on the exceptional, and emphatically on the utilitarian, which justifies medical science. In filling the pages it has pleased us to observe how much can be said with comparatively few words.

Illustration has been carefully planned, adhering to a ratio of almost a picture a page. The illustrations were selected from a considerable collection, and we intend them individually to be useful and pertinent. Dr. Herman Pinkus provided us with an exceptionally fine lot depicting normal anatomy; we are most grateful to him. Dr. H. J. Parkhurst, Dr. Clyde Cummer, Dr. George Miller MacKee, and many others to whose generosity figures are accredited, have given us the use of their photographs. Many an illustration has been taken from a journal article, the exact source being noted within the title for convenience of reference.

Dr. Harold Cole revised our chart for antisyphilitic treatment.

More than seven hundred fifty volume and page citations of pertinent literature are incorporated in the text, so that greater detail and original contributions may readily be studied according to desire or assignment.

RICHARD L. SUTTON
RICHARD L. SUTTON, JR.

# HANDBOOK
# OF
# DISEASES OF THE SKIN

by

**RICHARD L. SUTTON, M.D.**

Emeritus Professor of Dermatology and Syphilology,
University of Kansas Medical School

and

**RICHARD L. SUTTON, JR., M.D.**

Associate Professor of Dermatology and Syphilology,
University of Kansas Medical School

*WITH 1057 ILLUSTRATIONS*

ST. LOUIS
THE C. V. MOSBY COMPANY
1949

52

# PREFACE

The brevity and practicality at which I aimed in our *Synopsis of Diseases of the Skin* are also aims of this volume, which is intended to supply a text useful to medical students, practitioners, and specialists in dermatology. The medical student who knows a good deal of what is presented here in larger type will be better instructed in dermatology and syphilology than most medical students are. Practitioners seeking help in the interpretation and management of a case will profit from the illustrations, the prescriptions, and some of the material in smaller type. The scholar will find the volume comprehensive, for I have held to the policy of at least mentioning almost everything, and have included many thousands of bibliographic entries which enable one to find one's way about in the specialistic literature. These may be welcome even to the dermatologist certified as learned, whose memory, however disciplined, is unlikely to bear the burden of retaining everything at all times. This *Handbook* is more complete than our *Synopsis* and is less voluminous than the fourth edition of our *Introduction to Dermatology.*

Reviews of previous books of ours have received earnest deliberation, and the constructive criticisms have been adopted where they have not conflicted with the necessarily limited size of the book, or with each other, or with my desires. That I have colored the pages with personal views will please some readers and annoy others whose tastes or convictions differ from mine.

The order of presentation has been altered, with causation the principal guide to classification in the hope that it will appear logical to nondermatologists, who have tended with justification to think of dermatology as having possessed hitherto, to some extent, a viewpoint and language set apart from those of other sciences. I persist in wishing "to tie descriptions and concepts of disorders of the skin with general medicine and biology," as I wrote in 1938 in the preface of the tenth edition of our *Diseases of the Skin.*

Illustrations, numbering in excess of a thousand, have been carefully selected, trimmed, placed, and titled, their legends in appropriate instances giving the author and journal of their original publication.

References, abbreviated to their minimal consumption of space, have been incorporated within the textual material, where a reader can learn quickly to skip them or an investigator can use them immediately to find sources and elaborations of thoughts which have been trimmed, like the illustrations, to their essentials. Abbreviations of bibliographic references are on pages xi, ff.

The index should be pointed out as a source of a variety of information and guidance, especially under such titles as "Disease," "Prescription," "Syndrome," and "Test."

I would call attention to the technic of the treatment of contact dermatitis by elimination of all possible causes so that the patient is soon relieved, subsequently identifying the actual cause by systematic increment of the patient's chemical environment. This is original and effective. A practical technic is presented of detecting ingested allergens for the relief of urticaria, for which I am indebted to my associate, Bernard H. Winston, M.D. The section on syphilis is consistent with the literature available through the time of completing the galley proof. The presentation of acne vulgaris as a pustular lipidosis has been modified only in details after twelve years of application have failed to disturb my belief in the veracity of my views on its interpretation and treatment. Psychosomatic aspects of dermatology have received consideration. Disturbances of growth comprise a chapter which pleases me.

Hermann Pinkus, M.D., supplied us with beautiful photomicrographs of normal adult and fetal skin, and largely from his collection is drawn the noteworthy illustrative material of the chapters on Anatomy and Embryology.

Debts to others have been given meticulous acknowledgment throughout the text. I would also acknowledge indebtedness and express gratitude to many individuals who personally have helped me. Charles R. Rein, M.D., contributed expositions of the technic of serologic tests for syphilis. E. V. Allen, M.D., allowed me to reprint material from *Peripheral Vascular Diseases* by himself and collaborators. Oswaldo G. Costa, M.D., L. Halberstaedter, M.D., Harry M. Robinson, M.D., Harry M. Robinson, Jr., M.D., and Edward A. Gall, M.D., are among those whom I wish also to thank for pictures. Stephen Epstein, M.D., reviewed the section on staphylococcic infections in the skin. Bernard H. Winston, M.D., Norman D. Asel, M.D., Herbert Siesener, M.D., Frank Dwyer, M.D., Jeannette Carter, Ph.D., Rosellen Kissinger, R.N., Corinne Gallup, Hazel Hill, and Nadine Houston protected me from avoidable pressure of medical practice, relief from which was essential to the accomplishment of medical writing. Miss Hill indefatigably transformed manuscript from illegible to legible form. Dr. Winston painstakingly sought out with me the typographic errors in the page proof. Miss Opal Woodruff, Librarian, University of Kansas Medical Center, and Mr. Park Crawford, Acting Librarian, Jackson County Medical Society, gave me expert and cheerful assistance.

The advisory capacity of Richard L. Sutton, Sr., has continued since his retirement in 1935 from medical writing and in 1940 from medical practice. His influence on the manner of thinking herein exemplified is more significant than would have been his contribution of a factual trifle here and there. His senior authorship is to be acknowledged, for he caused me to inherit a book, which is a responsibility, and he taught me to try to cure people.

RICHARD L. SUTTON, JR.

411 Alameda Road
The Country Club Plaza
Kansas City 2, Missouri

# DISEASES

# OF THE SKIN

By RICHARD L. SUTTON, Jr., A.M., M.D., F.R.S. (Edin.)
CHAIRMAN OF THE DEPARTMENT OF DERMATOLOGY
UNIVERSITY OF KANSAS MEDICAL CENTER

*ELEVENTH EDITION*
*WITH 1972 ILLUSTRATIONS*

THE C. V. MOSBY COMPANY
ST. LOUIS 1956

# PREFACE TO ELEVENTH EDITION

*Diseases of the Skin* has been modernized to accord with medical literature through the date of closing the galley proof. It is comprehensive, yet condensed. It aims primarily at usefulness. The illustrations, 1,972 in number, are an atlas wherein all ordinary and many extraordinary dermatoses may be identified. The book includes features of a dictionary and an encyclopedia. It is a guide to the maze of what may be found, if one knows where to look, in an extensive medical library. It is a systematization of what is known about its subject, written from the viewpoint of a practicing physician who is inquisitive.

"The scholar will find the volume comprehensive," I wrote in the preface of our *Handbook of Diseases of the Skin* in 1949, "for I have held to the policy of at least mentioning almost everything and have included many thousands of bibliographic entries which enable one to find one's way about in the specialistic literature. These may be welcome, even to the dermatologist certified as learned, whose memory, however disciplined, is unlikely to bear the burden of retaining everything at all times. . . Reviews of previous books of ours have received earnest deliberation, and the constructive criticisms have been adopted where they have not conflicted with the necessarily limited size of the book, or with each other, or with my desires. . ."

The order of presentation here, as in the *Handbook,* uses causation as the principal guide to classification, "in the hope that it will appear logical to nondermatologists, who have tended with justification to think of dermatology as having possessed hitherto, to some extent, a viewpoint and language set apart from those of other sciences. I persist in wishing 'to tie descriptions and concepts of disorders of the skin with general medicine and biology,' as I wrote in 1938 in the preface of the tenth edition."

The utilization of page space has been painstaking. I put half of the words onto two-thirds of the page area available and used 8-point type for material of secondary importance, as I did in the *Handbook.* To print the book in 10 point only would necessitate publishing it in two volumes. A reader may merit sympathy when he peruses material set in small type, I know; but reading it is easier than writing it, and printing it, more informative than omitting it. The chapter on diseases due to fungi would in itself make a book of 200 pages. That on malformations and neoplasms would make one of 500 pages with 486 illustrations. I have incorporated more material on the psychosomatic aspects of dermatology than is to be found on the psychosomatic aspects of the whole field of psychiatry in a well-known, popular and massive volume on that specialty. The 6-point bibliographies total over 5,000 lines of type and present thumbnail abstracts of thousands of articles.

Outstanding are the illustrations. Hermann Pinkus, M.D., supplied for the *Handbook* a magnificent collection of photomicrographs of normal adult and embryonic cutaneous tissues. I am indebted here, too, for his normal material. Dr. Pinkus prepared for this edition a handsome collection of photomicrographs of abnormal tissues, which are used to illustrate the chapter on Pathology. Credit for numerous excellent illustrations is due Drs. J. Lamar Calloway, O. G. Costa, Clyde L. Cummer, Robert N. Andrade, Emanuel Muskatblit, John Belisario and F. Ronchese. The clinical pictures of Drs. Calloway, Costa, Cummer, Andrade and Ronchese are scattered throughout the book. Those of

Dr. Belisario are in the section on Carcinoma. Those of Dr. Muskatblit, showing fungi and diseases caused by them, are of unusual excellence, as are also those so generously given to me for previous editions by Drs. George M. Lewis and Mary Hopper. The privilege of taking what I desired from *Oral Pathology* by Kurt Thoma and from *Skin Manifestations of Internal Disorders* by Kurt Wiener deserves especial acknowledgment. To Dr. Gustav Riehl I am indebted for many fine illustrations of cutaneous tuberculosis, to Dr. S. William Becker for a group showing the histology of nevi and melanomas, and to Drs. Duncan Poth and J. J. Zoon for groups showing kerato-acanthoma.

The bibliography as a whole consists of that which is incorporated in the text plus that which is postscripted to the particular section. This latter material contains what I did not fit into the text yet desired to mention. To many such references I have added a word or two, identifying them, refreshing the memory of one who has read them before, or giving some idea of the content to one who has not.

In judging the ideas that are quoted so profusely in the text, one should note the dates of the references; I was aware of them.

Documentation can be accomplished in only a few ways. Superscript numbers and corresponding terminal references are not practicable. Footnotes are hopelessly confining when one intends to re-edit a book, for classifications change in fifty years. Finally, why insert "(Smith, 1951)" and oblige the reader to look to the end of the topic for the bibliographic reference, when one can insert "(Smith: Lancet 2: 1020, 1951)" and have done with it? I asked many friends for advice about styles of documentation and learned that two-thirds of them preferred mine, and four-fifths of them considered mine either preferable or acceptable.

Credit within the text, the bibliographies, and the titles of illustrations is everywhere carefully given. For that, too, which is original, the source is indicated. My opinions are nowhere hard to find. I remember with gratitude a review by a man who approved of my expression of personal opinions; that man will like this book. I claim some originality in paragraphs to be found hereinafter on several topics: the treatment of contact dermatitis; the interpretation and treatment of acne; the histologic and clinical understanding of early epidermoid carcinoma; the interpretation of autoeczematization and its relation to hypoproteinemia; what to do about chronic dermatitis of undetermined etiology, especially when it affects the hands; a certain hyperkeratotic form of volar dermatitis; the treatment of prurigo nodularis and of calcinosis universalis; *Microsporum canis* infection of the finger tips; *Gaffkya tetragena* infections of the skin; what I have chosen to call "Summertime pityriasis of the elbows and knees"; summer acne of the extremities; and apocrine cysts of the scalp, which I have not seen described elsewhere.

Dr. Charles R. Rein wrote the section on Serology of Syphilis, as he did for the tenth edition and the *Handbook*.

Dr. F. Stanley Morest read the section on Peripheral Vascular Disorders. The improvements he recommended attest to his extensive and effectual knowledge of this subject.

The galley proof on Leprosy was read by Rolla R. Wolcott, M.D., Medical Director, U. S. Public Health Service Hospital, Carville, Louisiana, and the material was conformed with his invaluable criticisms. I am grateful to Hermann Pinkus, M.D., further, for he graciously pointed to certain corrections desirable in the page proof of the chapter on Anatomy, to Walter C. Lobitz, Jr., M.D., who did this for the chapter on Physiology and the section on Diseases of the Sweat Glands, and to Sloan Wilson, M.D., who did it for the section on Purpura. What imperfections remain are not the fault of these kind friends.

Gilbert E. Ryder, M.D., for whom I am presently preceptor under the American Board of Dermatology and Syphilology, read all of the page proof with me. There is not a "dilatation" in the book, other than this one, not a "therapeutic armamentarium." We corrected an occasional misspelling in a direct quotation in order to avoid an uncharitable "[sic]."

The index is pointed out as a source of a variety of information and guidance, especially under such titles as "Disease," "Prescription," "Syndrome," and "Test."

Abbreviations of references are listed on p. xix, ff., preceding the text.

Many have asked me how such a book as this is made. One obviously depends on the publications of others, to which one's own observations and opinions are added. Among the requisites are time, experience in the practice of medicine (to which I have by now devoted some twenty-five years) and a generous measure of stubbornness. Of writing a book, Winston Churchill said, "To begin with, it is a toy and an amusement. Then it becomes a mistress, then a master; then it becomes a tyrant. Finally, when you are reconciled to your servitude, you kill the monster."

I have worked during morning hours, protected from every kind of interruption by teammates, who have occasionally been obliged to tax their consciences in defending me from people who itch. During 1953 a partnership with Norman D. Asel, M.D., was established. To our comfortable and satisfying relationship I am indebted for many hours that could have been granted me in no other way. I am grateful for the cheerful and efficient cooperation of Miss Margaret Egy, my patient secretary, skilled not only in orthography and syntax but also in getting along with a moody man, and of Mrs. Betty Standke, Miss Mildred Young, Mrs. Corinne Gallup, Mrs. Margaret Lynch, and Mr. Robert Sauvan.

Systematic reading is required. For years I have abstracted onto 3 x 5 file cards everything appertaining to dermatology that crossed my desk. These are cast alphabetically by subject matter. In abstracting, I record that which appears to add to my own knowledge. Most articles contain, of what I want, less than enough to crowd one side of a file card. The content of an exceptional essay may oblige me to use several sentences. One that I could not condense much, for example, was that of Bedford Shelmire (J 113: 1085, 1939) on dermatitis due to plants, of which I quoted whole paragraphs (p. 154). Some articles condense to nothing at all.

My descriptions of "a disease" frequently take the form of a reference to the original recognition of the entity, a statement of what may be called its average manifestations, and then several case references suggesting range, variability or extremes of its potentialities. The mention of rare, odd or curious instances helps, I imagine, in formulating a concept of the condition. Also, to me these are interesting.

In revising a description of a disease, I put together the pertinent group of file cards, some of which are cross references, like fragments of a mosaic. Sometimes an article is quoted with respect to only a fraction of its content, particularly if it covers a certain facet of the subject nicely, and I cite other articles appropriate to document other facets.

Here and there I quote a statement or hypothesis that is patently absurd, although not to its originator. I have done this to dispel ennui and to exemplify some of the contemporary "thinking" that is not critical (see Asher: BMJ 2: 460, 1954). Yet to me there is apparent in what I have written some mellowing with maturity as evidenced by a recently acquired lack of conviction that certain opinions of others are wrong or that opinions of mine are right. Credit has evolved into credibility, certitude into wonder, faith into hope. Thus where I have expressed my views, I may have antagonized fewer individuals in this edition than formerly, and in places I have actually avoided disputation.

Pertinent is a quotation you will enjoy, from an obscure source my father and I happened upon. John Smith, M.D.E., Coll. Med. Lond. Cand., published *King Solomon's Portraiture of Old Age Wherein Is Contained a Sacred*

*Anatomy Both of Soul and Body,* in 1666. His "Epistle to the Reader," in contrast with what was then customary, was not devoted to flattery of a patron. John Smith, whatever might have been his now quaint ideas on "sacred anatomy of soul and body," was a man one would like to know, and his preface, cold from his pen these 290 years, pleases me (I wish I could tell him so): "Whosoever thou are into whose hands this Paraphrase may fall, know that the Author of it is not near enough any Nobleman to put it into his hands, nor hath he face enough to call at a distance; but could he do both, yet know also he would do neither; for he desireth not that anything either of others or of his own should be patronized beyond its own native worth, And is himself willing . . . that all the shame that is due to the ill managing of this good Subject should return upon his own pate. . . ."

Those to whom Senior can be only a tradition may wish to become acquainted with the man who initiated this book in 1916 and put it through eight editions single-handed by 1931. My father was friendly, communicative, buoyant, desirous of approval. When he became famous, he enjoyed it immensely. He was the antithesis of colorless, being uninhibited in expressing vivid views. His contemporaries do not forget him; he did not bore them. Fishing and hunting were coequal with medicine in his enthusiasm, and he covered the earth in his travels. Vast numbers of persons from all walks of life adored him. Few have filled the hours of a lifetime so full. Obituaries were written by Harold N. Cole (ADS 66: 424, 1952), John Belisario (Austral JDermat 1: 263, 1953), and myself in the Yearbook (1951-1952) of the Royal Society of Edinburgh.

My father retired in 1940 to devote himself to the hunting and fishing he so dearly loved. His health did not long remain good. While new editions had been his almost biennial habit, the eleventh remained only an ambition for a number of years. The necessity for revising our *Introduction to Dermatology* in 1941, and my entry into military service not long thereafter, caused delay. By 1949 I had prepared our *Handbook* for publication, after which I again gave thought to tackling "the Big Red Book." Senior's death in May of 1952 made the task seem impossible. He had the ability to make hard work easy and to revivify when energy flagged. His decisions were instant and generally right, and his capacity for turning out work commanded the respect, even the awe, of those who knew him.

In the preface of the first edition of *Diseases of the Skin,* published in 1916 with 916 pages and 701 illustrations, my father said: "The present volume is the outgrowth of several years of study along this particular line and is an attempt to present the entire subject of dermatology in a comprehensive and, at the same time, concise manner. A treatise covering so broad a field . . . cannot well be based entirely on the personal knowledge and observations of any single individual. For this reason I have not hesitated to draw from the publications of other writers, selecting the material which I considered most appropriate. Every effort has been made to properly credit the ideas thus secured. . . . The majority of the therapeutic measures recommended are those which I have found useful and practicable in my own practice."

The second edition appeared in 1917, containing 1021 pages and 841 illustrations. The preface read, "The demand for a second edition at this time has given me opportunity to supply supplemental matter in a few instances, as well as to cover the important literature of the year 1916 and to eliminate a number of typographic and other minor errors. . . . I am deeply grateful to my friends and colleagues for the kind and generous reception accorded the first edition. . ."

The third edition, with 1084 pages and 921 illustrations, appeared in 1919. "While the war has had a deterrent effect upon the study of cutaneous medicine in general, it has added to our knowledge of the successful management of a few disorders, notably those due to animal parasites; and has developed a few new affections, such as occupation and traumatic dermatoses due to tetryl, dichlorethylsulphide and similar chemical irritants. . . . The gravity of syphilis as a social disease is becoming more evident each year, a fact to which attention has been called by the splendid contributions of William Allen Pusey, John H. Stokes, Loyd Thompson, H. H. Hazen, and other authorities. The important part played by focal infections in the causation of disorders of the skin is at last becoming generally recognized. I am indebted to many colleagues for valued suggestions and advice, and particularly to my friend, Dr. Charles J. White, of Boston, whose encouragement and example have been constant sources of inspiration during my entire dermatological career."

The fourth edition was published in 1921 with 1132 pages and 980 illustrations. "The clinical and serological study of syphilis continues to hold the attention of a large and able body of investigators, and the general public is at last beginning to appreciate the widespread prevalence and disastrous consequences of this malady. The researches of Ormsby and Mitchell, Charles J. White, Wende and Wilkinson, and others, on epidermophyton infection and its etiologic relationship to certain chronic inflammatory disorders of the skin, have served to call attention to an important field which has hitherto been sadly neglected in this country. . ."

The fifth edition, in 1923, contained 1214 pages and 1080 illustrations. "To one who has had a watchful finger on the pulse of dermatological literature for a decade and a half, the output for the past two years is as promising as it has been prolific. . . I am indebted to my son, Richard L. Sutton, Jr., for many of the photomicrographs. . ."

The sixth edition, in 1926, contained 1303 pages and 1158 illustrations. "Additional light is constantly being thrown on a number of cutaneous disorders, and while our therapeutic advances have not kept pace with the information gained along other lines, we at least are in position to combat the various mycotic disorders far more intelligently, if not more successfully, than we were a decade ago. . ."

The seventh edition appeared in 1928 with 1394 pages and 1248 illustrations. "Several recently discovered diseases have been introduced, the descriptions of some of the older ones rewritten, and the importance of others, such as certain of the occupational dermatoses, and those related to allergy, emphasized. An attempt has been made to discuss intelligibly the latest developments in cutaneous therapy, and to recommend those agents known to be reliable and practicable. . . In order to economize space, a considerable number of valuable references have had to be confined wholly to footnotes; otherwise the volume would soon become so bulky and unwieldy as to seriously impair its usefulness."

The eighth edition was published in 1931 with 1352 pages and 1301 illustrations. "Modern dermatological literature appears to grow by leaps and bounds. . . . It is essential that each new edition contain an easily accessible and complete record of all the authoritative reports that have appeared in the interval. This I have endeavored to do to the best of my ability, but even the most skilled of phraseological artists will experience difficulty in condensing and crystallizing the wisdom of a three thousand word masterpiece into the space of one or two brief sentences, and I must acknowledge that I am no literary Cellini. Scanning the completed task, no one realizes better than I how incompletely it fulfills the ideal."

The ninth edition, the first of Sutton and Sutton coauthorship, was published in 1935 with 1433 pages and 1321 illustrations. "Twenty years ago, when I began collecting material for the first edition of this work," Senior wrote, "little did I suspect that it would ever grow into the present ponderous volume. Had I done so, it is very probable that I should have tried to content myself with labors that demanded far less time and effort. A book of this sort is like a child; the author, an anxious and doting parent."

The tenth edition, a three-year labor of rewriting, appeared in 1939 with 1549 pages and 1473 illustrations. With emendations, it was reprinted in 1942 and again in 1943. We imagined that we had systematized the progressively increasing difficulty of reflecting current dermatology in such a fashion that future editions would be relatively easy to prepare. I wrote the preface that time: "In view of the favorable reception accorded the etiologic classification in the 1937 edition of our *Introduction to Dermatology,* and the tendency nowadays to inquire 'What is going on?' rather than 'What name is applicable to this manifestation?' the material has been arranged in a fashion radically different from that in the ninth edition. . . Descriptions of all significant entities, syndromes and concepts, and of many exotic, unusual, and even exceptional dermatoses have been incorporated. Emphasis is laid, however, on the purpose of practical medicine, which is to cure the ordinary patient of his ordinary complaints by scientific or by pragmatic means."

Quotations from prefaces of the past indicate that the endeavor to reflect contemporary medical thinking and practice involves a variety of problems. They are problems that become more and more challenging as one measures the capacity of a human being against the quantity of dermatologic science (and fiction) that appears in print.

RICHARD L. SUTTON, JR.

Kansas City, Missouri

# THE SKIN

## *A Handbook*

RICHARD L. SUTTON, Jr.

A.M., M.D., F.R.S. (Edin.)

*Clinical Professor of Medicine (Dermatology), University of Kansas Medical Center; Consultant in Dermatology, University of Missouri Medical Center; Former Consultant Dermatoses Investigations Section, National Institute of Health, U. S. Public Health Service*

DOUBLEDAY & COMPANY, INC.
GARDEN CITY, NEW YORK

# PREFACE

My purpose is to provide a perspective of the skin in health and disease that is simple, clear and relatively comprehensive. The book is for any individual concerned with a skin problem of his own or of someone whose welfare is important to him.

The structure and function of the skin and its care and hygiene are described as well as abnormalities. Whoever has a skin problem can find material here that will help him understand it and quite possibly do something about it to his advantage.

Common diseases receive more consideration and rare ones less, while mentioning the unusual has seemed appropriate now and then. Acne, psoriasis, dermatitis due to irritants, and the early stages of skin cancer are among the subjects discussed at length. In the choice of what to include and the emphasis to apportion, no two authors would reach the same decisions. I have been guided by what I have learned in thirty years of practice.

The book consists of two parts. The first seven chapters are concerned with fundamentals; the remainder, with specific diseases, where "one gets down to cases." Diseases are classified by causes insofar as these are known. While the everyday language does not contain names for some of them, the vocabulary is that of Webster's New Collegiate Dictionary. When an inescapable technical word appears, its meaning is given. The index provides page references to definitions or explanations of unfamiliar words. Treatment suggested for each disease is contemporary and in accord with the plans systematically outlined in Chapter 7. Almost everything needed to carry out such self-medication as is recommended is in the "Household Remedies" list.

The book is suitable for dermatologists to recommend to some of their patients, I believe; and teachers, to their students of medicine, dentistry, and nursing.

I am grateful to the many people who have made the book possible and acknowledge especially my debt to patients with whom I have worked. Only from patients can one learn the varieties of their problems and the questions they ask and the ways of answering that give satisfaction.

Richard L. Sutton, Sr., M.D., employed me as his assistant after my preliminary medical training and educated me further. He let me help with revisions of his *Diseases of the Skin,* the first edition of which was published in 1916, and later turned the book over to me lock, stock, and barrel after he elected in 1940 to hunt and fish continually rather than as an avocation. The C. V. Mosby Company permitted me the use of material from the eleventh edition, published in 1956.

Norman D. Asel, M.D., formerly my partner and now Professor of Dermatology, University of Missouri Medical Center, allowed me to give to writing much energy I might have used in our collaborative medical practice. Our relationship without a cross word in seven years is a privileged memory. I am grateful to Mrs. Margaret Egy Lehr, my secretary, Mr. Robert L. Sauvan, microbiologist, Miss Mildred Young, Mrs. Jack E. Sproul, and Mrs. Lyle Metzdorf for their contributions to the expedition of our work and my peace of mind.

Credit is due David W. Robinson, M.D., Professor of Plastic Surgery, University of Kansas Medical Center, for help with paragraphs on the abrasive treatment of acne scars, and Marvin L. Bills, M.D., for a critique of the chapter on abnormalities of the psyche. The paragraphs on venomous bites accord with the counsel of Herbert L. Stahnke, Ph.D., Director, Poisonous Animals Research Laboratory, Arizona State University. Richard C. Wright, D.D.S., provided advice on several aspects of oral pathology. Richard N. Besley read the manuscript with the viewpoint of the medical student and made a number of helpful suggestions. Phillip H. Watkins, manager of the corner drugstore where I am most at home, and Henry C. O'Brien, Victor A. Miller, and Clarence A. Leonard, pharmacists, answered countless questions. George L. Heavilin, of the School of Hair Fashion and Cosmetology, was a source of useful information. Miss Edith Hodgson, medical artist, prepared the frontispiece, and her representation of the structure of the skin earned the approval of my friend, Hermann Pinkus, M.D., dermal pathologist. Mrs. Isabelle Taylor, editor, Doubleday and Company, encouraged a dissimulated preference for monosyllables. Norton Canfield, M.D., Professor of Otology, Yale University, a fraternity brother of medical school days, was instrumental in my undertaking the book.

RICHARD L. SUTTON, JR., M.D.

*Kansas City, Missouri*
*9 July 1961*

# THE PRACTITIONERS' DERMATOLOGY

*by*

Richard L. Sutton, Jr., M.D., F.R.S. (Edin.)
**Prairie Village, Kansas 66208**
*Clinical Professor Emeritus of Medicine (Dermatology)*
*University of Kansas Medical Center*
*Senior Consulting Clinical Professor of Medicine (Dermatology)*
*University of Missouri Medical Center*
*Adjunct Professor of Geosciences*
*University of Missouri–Kansas City*

*and*

Morris Waisman, M.D.
**Tampa, Florida 33602**
*Clinical Professor of Medicine (Dermatology) and*
*Clinical Professor of Pharmacology*
*University of South Florida College of Medicine*
*Adjunct Professor of Dermatology*
*University of Miami School of Medicine*

## PREFACE

When I was my father's junior employee forty-five years ago, I noted he occasionally said to a patient, pointing to his ponderous *Diseases of the Skin*, "I wrote that when I was young and foolish." Appreciative now of what he meant, and no longer young, and presumably less foolish than I used to be, I induced Morris Waisman to write this with me. He and I believe we have something to say.

Our book is intended especially for practitioners—family, internal medical, pediatric, dermatologic—and for medical students and recent graduates. We seek to clarify why one orders what one does rather than merely what to order. On the subject of clarity, parenthetically, we think that when a reader doesn't understand a sentence the writer didn't.

A medical book may be looked upon as a form of journalism, for it contains three kinds of writing: reportorial, intended as pure observation; editorial, as interpretation; and advertising. Dr. Waisman and I consider ourselves skilled at observing and interpreting, and we both have taught school and hold academic titles. Primarily, however, we are practitioners, and what we advertise is that practical medicine, while it differs from academic and investigative, is eminently worthy.

In choosing to collaborate, Dr. Waisman and I also considered the fact of our mutual respect and long friendship. It was originally our intention to say that we both believe everything in the book. When we actually set to work, we discovered that politics traditionally, marriage frequently, and coauthorship for sure make strange bedfellows. We somehow got around the astonishing first diametric disagreement and knew better how to deal with the next. Not all contentions could be compromised, we discovered, so in places we insert (W), which means Waisman thinks this, but Sutton doesn't, or (S), which means Sutton believes this, but Waisman doesn't. Commendations of x-ray therapy require no designation, you are to understand, for almost all are by Sutton, who is archaic enough to mourn the dying art of dermatologic radiotherapy and irreverent enough to disbelieve most of the clamor of the fruit-fly cognoscenti. After many months of collaboration, Dr. Waisman and I are convinced that no reviewer will say anything worse about some of our notions than we already have. I do wish to say I think only a few (W)'s as evil as Dr. Waisman thinks many (S)'s are—conviction being somehow inversely proportionate to age. Apparent to me also is a harrowing feature of this venture: married 39 years, I have nevertheless not hitherto been so often told I was wrong by someone who so often was right. Except about x-ray therapy. In general (W) connotes views that are conservative, party-line, and safe, and I think I would let him treat me. So we invite old friends to read us for fun and take sides in the disputes.

On the other hand, there are many things we both believe, and when we concur perhaps what we say is true. But the medical science that stays true for a long time is uncommon stuff. Look, for example, at classification. Etiologic classification was new in dermatology when I devised the 1939 edition of Sutton and Sutton's *Diseases of the Skin.* Erasmus Wilson tried in 1842, but he mistook pathology for etiology, being (naturally) a prisoner of the cultural climate. For thirty-five years I have believed morphologic classification naive and sterile, as unsophisticated as an idea that acne pustules and furuncles are really not much different.

With mature dermatologic scholarship, Sir Archibald Gray in his essay, "The Founders of Modern Dermatology," discussed Willan's morphologic approach (*Transactions of the St. John's Hospital Dermatological Society,* Autumn, 1955). Where, one asks, is the morphologist when he would comprehend contact dermatitis? This kind of disease is not to be found, it is interesting to note, in the 1572 *De Morbis Cutaneis* of Hieronymus Mercurialis. The dermatitis may be pink, blistery, leathery, fissured, but still *venenata* ("due to poison")—unless it is impetiginous, or atopic, or all three. In our discourse on the principles of treatment (Chapter 6) we give general solutions for the problems of how to deal with the standard etiologic kinds of diseases and, in particular, what to do when the cause is not known: you systematically peel off each of the known kinds of causes —and so their effects—one by one until naked before your eyes, so to speak, lies what has not been fixed yet. Empirical, practical, effective. The morphologist cannot do this. The practitioner must.

Not to be found elsewhere are several other original notions, such as our identification of a relationship between too-hot baths and Schamberg's disease, our concern for what makes the skin irritable as well as for what irritates it, our observation that the painful nodule of the ear is simply a pressure sore, our often successful use in mucous retention cyst of the lip of an intracutaneous injection of triamcinolone acetonide, our exposition of the cause and cure of solenonychia, our eradication of dilated pore and hypertrophic fat gland with single doses of x-ray therapy, and our recognition of the palpable warmth of the active lesion in morphea.

Throughout our book, we recognize that the patient is not skin plus some other things. On separating skin from a human being, one has only a hide of low economic value and a carcass such as might be found on the littoral of Bering Strait. What the physician works with is greater than the sum of its parts.

It is a pleasure to acknowledge indebtedness. Our illustrations, collected over some seven decades, represent the masters of classic dermatologic photography—Grover Wende, Howard Fox, George M. MacKee, Samuel Sweitzer, and Richard L. Sutton, Sr., for example—as well as younger artists, J. Lamar Callaway, Francesco Ronchese, and Oswaldo G. Costa among the many. Credit is given unless the source was Waisman or a Sutton. More than 600 pictures are published, and they are not numbered, which is a novelty in a medical book, and I do not know the exact total, but they are good pictures. That is to say, they would stand up pretty well, most of them, without legends. Some legends convey information not put elsewhere, thereby avoiding repetition.

References are of no use to a reader without a library, nor to a reader with one since he will be able to find articles more recent than those to which we can refer. Therefore bibliographies are omitted. A look about in a medical library will do no doctor harm, and a student assigned the task might even think it entertaining to hunt up where we got our information. As Logan Clendening, founder of the

History of Medicine Library of the University of Kansas, said to me: "Young man, if you don't know what a library is for, your father wasted a hell of a lot of money." Of course Dr. Waisman and I are aware that we originated an exceedingly small fraction of our material and are immeasurably in debt to innumerable colleagues, contemporary and antecedent.

We have received and appreciate the enthusiastic, expert, and dedicated cooperation of Ernest Zelenak, Lynne Nicholson, and Loretta Franklin Lumelleau, in particular, and all the others of the team of Yorke Medical Books, our publisher. Rachel (Mrs. Morris) Waisman contributed the laborious part of casting the index.

Richard L. Sutton, Jr.

4121 West 83rd Street
Prairie Village, Kansas 66208

23 May 1974

# Nonmedical Books
## TITLE PAGES AND PREFACES

# AN AFRICAN HOLIDAY

BY

RICHARD L. SUTTON, M.D., LL.D.

Fellow of the Royal Geographical Society of Great Britain

*With 102 Original Illustrations*

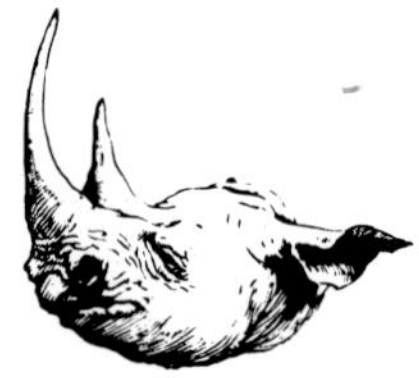

ST. LOUIS

THE C. V. MOSBY COMPANY

1924

# Preface

ALL GOOD sportsmen eventually go to Africa. If not in this life, then, as a sort of reward of merit, in the next. For this, the book shelf is largely to blame. I had no idea of the widespread popularity of Henry M. Stanley's great literary masterpiece until after I had begun a series of lectures, on my return home. In the majority of instances, it was this famous explorer who had first planted the seeds of desire, to be nourished and stimulated later by the fireside perusal of the inimitable tales of William Cotton Oswell and Gordon Cumming, Sir Samuel Baker and Frederick Selous, Colonel Patterson and our own Carl Akeley. In recent years, the marvellous pictures made by Mr. and Mrs. Martin Johnson have done much to arouse new interest regarding this fascinating and little-known country.

An African shooting trip nowadays is a comparatively simple affair. Given time, inclination, and a little means, it can be easily and safely undertaken by any able-bodied man between the ages of sixteen and sixty-five.

I wish to express my thanks to the civil and military authorities of Kenya Colony for the many courtesies extended to us during our visit. I am particularly indebted to Captain K. L. T. Caldwell, of the Game Department, and to the Customs officials at

Mombasa and at Nairobi. These gentlemen did everything in their power to render our trip as free as possible from worry and inconvenience.

Mr. Oscar Thomason, Acting Vice Consul at Nairobi, aided us in many ways. We are also under obligation to Dr. R. W. Burkitt, the eminent surgeon, to Mr. R. F. Mayer, the brilliant and affable editor of the "East African Standard," and to Mr. Robert Boyd, of the "Farmer's Journal."

Our greatest debt, however, is to a representative soldier-settler, Major Sidney Armstrong, of Nonyouki. He was our first and best friend in Africa, and we shall always feel grateful to him for his kindness and generous hospitality.

A few of the pictures are made from photographs taken by my brother, and by our white hunter, Alan Black, and two, those of the charging elephant and of the giraffe, by our first guide, Captain G. H. R. Hurst. Of our friends and acquaintances in America, we are most indebted to Mr. Carl Akeley, and his associate, Mr. James Clark, of the American Museum of Natural History; Mr. Stewart Edward White; Mr. Huston Wyeth, the widely known sportsman, of St. Joseph, Missouri; Mr. Jo Zach Miller, III, of Kansas City; and Commander Fred Robinson, and Mr. Harper, of the Cunard Lines.

Nearly all of the included material was first published, as a series of letters, in the "Kansas City Star," and I am under obligation to this newspaper for courteous permission to use it here.

There is an old Arab saying that "He who drinks of Africa's fountains will return to quench his thirst again," and I fear that it is based on fact. The long, hard treks soon are forgotten, the memories of painful and disagreeable incidents quickly fade, and one remembers only the kindliness and hospitality of a simple and primitive people, and the quiet peace of the everlasting hills.

Here the ambitious course of Empire is halted by natural barriers, and even inexorable Time seems almost at a standstill. No one has epitomized the situation more beautifully than Cecil John:

> "Yours is the wild and lovely land
> Untouched by human blight;
> Yours is the wilderness' last stand,
> Beauty's last desperate fight.
> Fever and tsetse and fierce sun—
> Without them you were soon undone!"

R. L. S.

Kansas City, March, 1924.

# TIGER TRAILS
# IN SOUTHERN ASIA

BY

RICHARD L. SUTTON, M.D., Sc.D., LL.D., F.R.S. (Edin.)

Fellow of the Royal Geographical Society; Professor of Dermatology,
University of Kansas; Special Representative, Department
of Natural History, University of Missouri

*With 115 Original Illustrations*

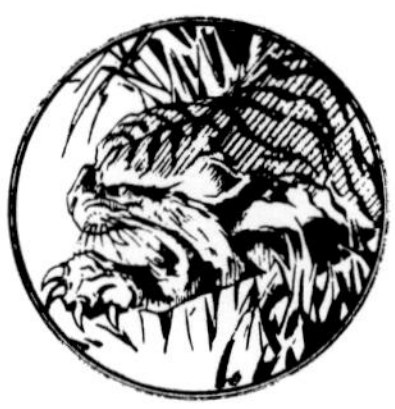

ST. LOUIS

THE C. V. MOSBY COMPANY

1926

# Foreword

This little volume is not an authoritative treatise on tigers. In reality, it is a compilation of a series of notes made on a trip which originally was planned as a vacation, but which ultimately developed into a sort of endurance test. While the book contains some first-hand information, painfully gleaned, it was written entirely for pleasure, and should be read, if read at all, for the same reason.

It has been suggested that many big game hunters take themselves and their sport entirely too seriously. To them, every lion is a man-eater, every elephant a rogue, or a huge, devil-may-care tusker, thirsting for human gore. Aside from the rhinoceros, whose mercurial temperament is probably due as much to a morbid and moronic inquisitiveness as to innate ferocity, man-hunting animals are rare, and an unarmed native of Tanganyika, Cambodia or Assam is in far less danger on his own native heath than a healthy and well-trained Kansas Citian would be while dodging motor cars in Petticoat Lane.

There are of course a few hardships to be met, and difficulties to be overcome, but these should only whet the appetite, and whether you are crouching behind a tiny grass screen, waiting for a tiger, or plodding along beneath a red-hot sun, trying to get within gunshot of a big bull elephant, or lounging on the sandy bank of a tropical river, at the end of a perfect day, you love it all, and afterward you will return to the hard pavements, and the clanging street cars, and the insistent telephone, and the thousand and one other irritating perplexities of city life, a saner and a wiser, if not a happier and a better man.

I am indebted to many friends and acquaintances for advice and assistance on the present expeditions. Mr. Jo Zach Miller III, secured for me letters of introduction from Mr. W. B. Walker, of the Standard Oil Company of New York, to various representatives of the Company in the Far East, and at Hongkong, Singapore, and, particularly, Saigon, I am indebted to these splendid young men for a multitude of kindnesses.

Mr. Harry Pethick, of the Hongkong office, especially was very generous, and I am under obligation to him for the excellent photographs of Angkor, while Mr. Acton Poulet, who is the most influential, as well as the most popular, oil man in all Asia, did everything in his power to make our stay in Indo-China a pleasant as well as a profitable one. We had a mutual friend in Mr. Frank Crowell Baker, of Kansas City, and this, together with the fact that Mr. Poulet was educated at the University of Kansas and at Yale, and is a fraternity brother of Mr. Waddell, made us feel that while visiting him and his charming and beautiful sister, Mrs. Horace Dickinson, we were with home folks.

To Judge James E. Goodrich, Chairman of the Board of Curators of the University of Missouri, and to President Stratton Brooks, I am indebted for the temporary appointment on the Faculty of my beloved Alma Mater.

Through the kindness of Senator James A. Reed, Sir Esme Howard, the British Ambassador to the United States, became interested in our plans for visiting India, and had the little expedition been a personal one, his Excellency could not have done more to further its success. Throughout our stay, their Excellencies, the Earl of Lytton, Governor of Bengal, and Sir John Kerr, K.C.S.I., Governor of Assam, did everything in their power to aid us.

In the chapter on Tribes and Castes, I have drawn freely from the published work of Russell, Crooke, Fraser, Westermarck, Risley, Senart, Lyall, Purdon, and, particularly, Crawford. The statistical records I have taken from the Indian Census Reports for 1901, 1911, and 1921.

Nearly all of the included material was first published, as a series of letters, in "The Kansas City Star," and I am under obligation to this newspaper for courteous permission to use it here.

The chapter on Transportation and Equipment has been added for the information and benefit of brother sportsmen.

R. L. S.

Kansas City, May, 1926.

# THE LONG TREK

## Around the World with Camera and Rifle

BY

RICHARD L. SUTTON, M.D., Sc.D., LL.D., F.R.S. (Edin.)

Fellow of the Royal Geographical Society; Member of the French Geographical Society; Professor of Dermatology, University of Kansas

*With more than two hundred illustrations, from photographs made by the author*

AND BY

RICHARD L. SUTTON, JR., A.M., B.Sc., M.D.

Fellow of the Royal Geographical Society

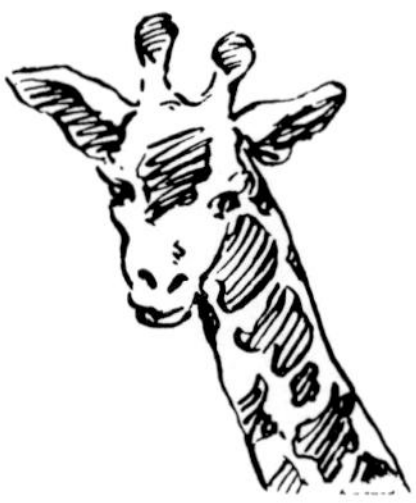

ST. LOUIS

THE C. V. MOSBY COMPANY

1930

82

# Preface

This brief narrative is really the story of a birthday party.

Many years before, I had promised my young son that when he attained his majority, provided his college and university records warranted it, we would indulge in a real celebration.

For more than a decade we had hunted and fished together in the Middle West, in the West, in Texas, in Mexico, in Florida, and in Canada; consequently if the "party" was to be a really worth-while one, newer and more interesting territory must be found.

Our first thought was the Pamirs, in Russian Turkestan, with side trips to Africa, and probably to Borneo; but some of my medical confreres ruled otherwise, and when we found that we must stick to lower latitudes, we selected East Africa, Sumatra, and Indo-China.

I had previously shot in Kenya, so we decided to try Tanganyika.

Earlier experience, in India and in other parts of Southern Asia, had convinced me that the best tiger shooting in the world is to be had in Laos and Annam. We had long been in touch with Mons. F. J. Defosse, of Suoi Kiet, whom I consider the premier white hunter of the world, and he and his son, Louis, kindly placed their services at our disposal.

Fortunately, both of us are enthusiastic photographers as well as hunters, and this field proved one of our greatest sources of pleasure. While we failed to discover any strange and beautiful lakes in the neighborhood of Nairobi or in the immediate vicinity of Archer's old boma, and did not succeed in killing a single elephant with bow and arrow, we did endeavor to behave ourselves as sportsmen should, abstained from chasing wart hogs with a motor car, and made a host of interesting new acquaintances and friends.

To many of these we are indebted for courtesies and favors. Mr. William Brown Robertson, district officer of Mbulu, was extremely kind to us. Captain Minnery, chief game ranger of northern Tanganyika, allowed us to take photographs in Ngoro Ngoro Crater; Mr. C. M. Clark, the chief customs officer at Tanga, showed us every courtesy. Mr. McQuade and his associates, of the Mombasa Customs, gave us much helpful assistance and advice, and several of the officials of the Kenya-Uganda Railway and Boat Lines personally saw that we had the best of service.

Of the old friends who aided us, their name is legion. Many years ago Senator James A. Reed was so kind as to interest the British Ambassador, the Right Honorable Sir Esme Howard, K.C.B., in one of my expeditions. Since then I have become indebted to His Excellency for a score of invaluable favors. He has always done everything within his power to make my scientific excursions to the far corners of the earth a success, and I owe him much that I can never repay.

To Senator William E. Borah, chairman of the committee on foreign affairs, likewise, we are heavily indebted. The credentials which he gave us proved of great value, not only in Africa, but at Singapore, Batavia, and in Indo-China as well.

Mr. W. B. Walker, of the Standard Oil Company, New York, generously gave me letters to representatives of his organization at Saigon and at Singapore, and I am under obligation to these gentlemen for their generous hospitality. Particularly is this true with respect to Mr. Acton Poulet, of Indo-China. He is the best known and most popular European business man in Southern Asia, and possesses enormous influence throughout the country.

Practically all of the material here included has previously appeared in *The Kansas City Star* and *The New York Times*, and I wish to thank the editors of these newspapers for their courtesy.

Mr. George Petroll, of the Hamburg-American Lines, saved us much time and trouble; the officials of the Deutsch-East African Steamship Company gave us special service and attention; and Captain Mory, of the "Mexico Maru," Osaka Shosen Kaisha, was so kind as to make us his personal guests during our stay in the Flowery Kingdom.

For two of the chapters, those entitled "Kiswahili" and "The Wambulu People," and for more than one half of the photographs, I am indebted to my son and associate, Dr. Richard L. Sutton, Jr.

R. L. S.

# AN ARCTIC SAFARI

## With Camera and Rifle in the Land of the Midnight Sun

BY

RICHARD L. SUTTON, M.D., Sc.D., LL.D., F.R.S. (Edin.)

Fellow of the Royal Geographical Society; Member of the French Geographical Society; Professor of Dermatology, University of Kansas

*With more than one hundred illustrations, made from photographs taken by the author*

AND BY

RICHARD L. SUTTON, JR., A.M., M.D.

AND

EMMY LOU SUTTON, F.R.G.S.

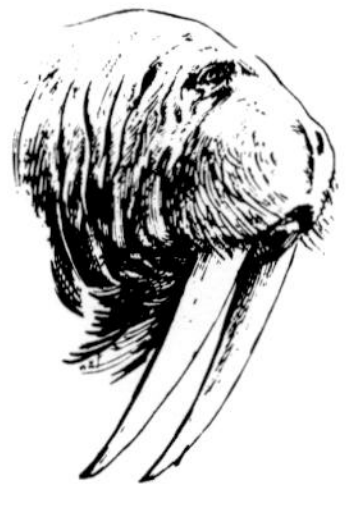

ST. LOUIS

THE C. V. MOSBY COMPANY

1932

# Preface

EACH year the big game fields of the world are narrowed. It seems only yesterday that we shot antelope on the Colorado plains. Today a wild pronghorn is almost a curiosity.

Big game and civilization simply do not mix. The motor car was the straw that broke the camel's back.

On my last visit to Kenya, a friend in the King's African Rifles decided that he would like to kill a lion. With a light truck and a sophisticated white hunter he left barracks one October morning. Sixty hours later, he was back, with two lions. During that period he had covered eight hundred miles! Even the sturdiest and most athletic of felines cannot deny a man like that.

The expedition described in the following pages was undertaken for educational purposes as well as for sport.

An old and dear friend, Vilhjalmur Stefansson, the eminent explorer, often had told us of the beauty and grandeur of the Far North. Few men can paint a better word picture than he who discovered the white Esquimaux, and families such as mine, already imbued with an inordinate love of the great outdoors, naturally have a very low sales resistance to any strange region which is so replete with thrills.

I have always been a great admirer of Norwegian seamen, and for that reason we decided to sail, if possible, from a Northern Scandinavian port.

Experienced friends directed us to the Bennett Travel Bureau, of Oslo and of New York, and it was through this splendid organization that we secured the motorship "Isbjorn," of which Konsul Gudlief Holmboe, of Tromsö, is the deservedly proud owner.

The "Isbjorn" is a sealer, and ice boat, and as staunch and seaworthy as she is graceful and beautiful. She proved ideal for our purpose.

Together with my wife, son and daughter, and a crew which consisted of seventeen sailors and an experienced woman cook, we left Tromsö in May, 1932. We had purposely started early in the season, and ours was the first boat to reach shooting territory that spring. While the ice proved very embarrassing at times, we were so fortunate as to secure a large number of photographs, and a full complement of trophies and specimens.

Of the many friends to whom we are indebted, Dr. Stefansson comes first. In fact, if it had not been for this intrepid explorer, and kindly philosopher, the trip would never have been undertaken. When we left him in New York, his parting gift was a huge bundle of well selected books on arctic travel. These volumes we found helpful as well as entertaining, and during our stay in the ice, all of them were read and reread many times.

Of the various Bennett representatives with whom we came in contact, and to the prospective traveler I will say that the word "Bennett" is an open sesame throughout the Northern Country, we are most indebted to I. Giaver-Krogh, of Oslo. Mr. Krogh was born in Tromsö, and for many years has fitted out shooting expeditions to Spitsbergen, Franz Josef Land, and Greenland. All of this vast experience was at our disposal, and I must say, to use a British expression, that he "did us well." I have shot all over the world, and never have I had such admirable service. Not only did he save us much time and trouble, but his kindly forethought added immeasurably to our personal comfort and happiness. We shall always be grateful to him and to his charming wife for their kindness and generosity.

The officials of the Norwegian America Line extended to us every courtesy. We are particularly indebted to the First Officer of the SS. "Bergensfjord," Captain Halver Halvarsen, for many courtesies. Captain Halvarsen is a former whaling skipper, with much experience in the Antarctic, and it was to his tender care that we entrusted our rare hooded seals on the return trip to America.

All of the included matter previously appeared in the *Kansas City Star,* and I am under obligation to the Editor of that newspaper for permission to use it here.

For the translation of that portion of Professor Qvigstad's monograph on Spitsbergen Place names, which appears in the Appendix, I am indebted to my friend and former shipmate, Mr. Ernst Sorensen of Tromsö.

R. L. SUTTON.

Kansas City, Missouri.
October, 1932.

# THE SILVER KINGS of ARANSAS PASS
## *and Other Stories*

*By*

RICHARD L. SUTTON, F. R. G. S.

Author of Tiger Trails in Southern Asia;
An African Holiday; An Arctic Safari;
The Long Trek, Around the World
With Camera and Rifle, etc.

THE BROWN-WHITE COMPANY
THIRTY-FIRST STREET AND GRAND AVENUE
KANSAS CITY, MISSOURI

# PREFACE

A distinguished British sportsman once said, "Two thirds of my life I give to the city. The other third belongs to me." I agree with this gentleman.

The material for this volume was collected in various parts of the world at odd moments, and I trust the reader may share some of the thrills and pleasures that were experienced by my companions and me on these little excursions into the wilds. The period covered is approximately twenty years, from 1917 to 1937.

The book was written for fun, and should be read, if read at all, for the same reason.

I am grateful to my friends, the Editors of Field and Stream, Outdoor Life, Sports Afield, and the National Sportsman for permission to republish the stories here.

R. L. S.

Kansas City, Mo.

# *Chapter Headings*

and other verse

RICHARD L. SUTTON
M.D., Sc.D., LL.D., F.R.S. (Edin.)

BROWN-WHITE-LOWELL PRESS
KANSAS CITY, MISSOURI

# PREFACE

This little book contains a number of short poems which have previously appeared in various of my shooting and travel stories, An African Holiday, Tiger Trails in Southern Asia, The Long Trek, An Arctic Safari, and The Silver Kings of Aransas Pass.

The Red Cross Aide verses were written while I was taking an enforced rest in a Texas hospital.

The slender volume has been published at the insistence of my wife and fishing partner, and is affectionately dedicated to her. I feel that any grandmother who can break a world's record on eighteen thread line is entitled to every consideration.

R. L. S.

Kansas City, Mo.

# PRELIMINARY PALEONTOLOGICAL SURVEY

of the

BEARPAW SHALE BORDERING THE FORT PECK RESERVOIR, MONTANA

Under Department of the Interior Antiquities Act

Permit 70-MT-050

Report to the Smithsonian Institution

for the Paleontological Institute

University of Kansas, Lawrence, Kansas

Prof. Curt Teichert, Director

by

Richard L. Sutton, Jr., M.D.

1970

This is one of three bound copies, for Curt Teichert, William D. Greene and Dale Noble, and Richard L. Sutton, Jr.

Richard L. Sutton, Jr., M.D.

411 Nichols Road

Kansas City, Mo. 64112

1 February 1971

The Secretary
Smithsonian Institution
Washington, D. C.

Dear Sir:

Pursuant to paragraph 9 of the Antiquities Act Permit 70-MT-050 issued by the Department of the Interior, I send you herewith in sextuplicate, and to the Departmental Consulting Archeologist, National Park Service, one copy, the report of a preliminary paleontological survey of the Bearpaw Shale bordering the Fort Peck Reservior, Montana, in general charge, Dr. Curt Teichert, Director, Paleontological Institute, University of Kansas, Lawrence, Kansas 66044, and in direct charge, the undersigned.

The report comprises the following 13 pages and 1 map:

a) Letter of transmittal, page 1

b) Narrative account of procedure, personnel, and experience, page 2

c) Comment, page 3

d) Report on referred fossils, by Dr. William A. Cobban, Paleontology and Stratigraphy Branch, Denver Laboratories, U.S.G.S., pages 4-6

e) Tabulation of identifications of fossils found in specific areas, page 7

f) Legends of 20 photographs, page 8

g) Photographs pertinent to the region and fossils found, pages 9-13

h) Marked map, Jordan, Montana, Geologic Survey, Washington, D. C. 1958-NS MR-2782.

Very truly yours,

Richard L. Sutton, Jr.

Richard L. Sutton, Jr., M.D.

RLS/bjp
CC: Departmental Consulting Archeologist
Department of the Interior
National Park Service
801 19th Street N.W. - Room 621
Washington, D.C. 20006

# THE MISSOURI RIVER

## The River Rat's Guide To Missouri River History and Folklore

Compiled by Cecil R. Griffith 1903-1970

Edited and Published By
Kenneth R. Canfield
and
Richard L. Sutton, Jr.
3203 West 83rd. Terr.
Leawood, Kans. 66206

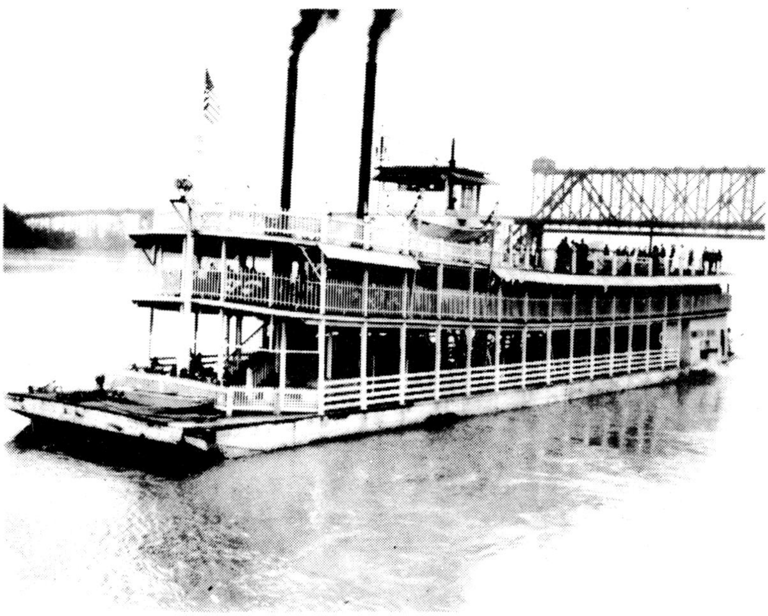

The John Heckman, Missouri River Steamboat, 1924

# Contents

# Portraits and Biographic Information

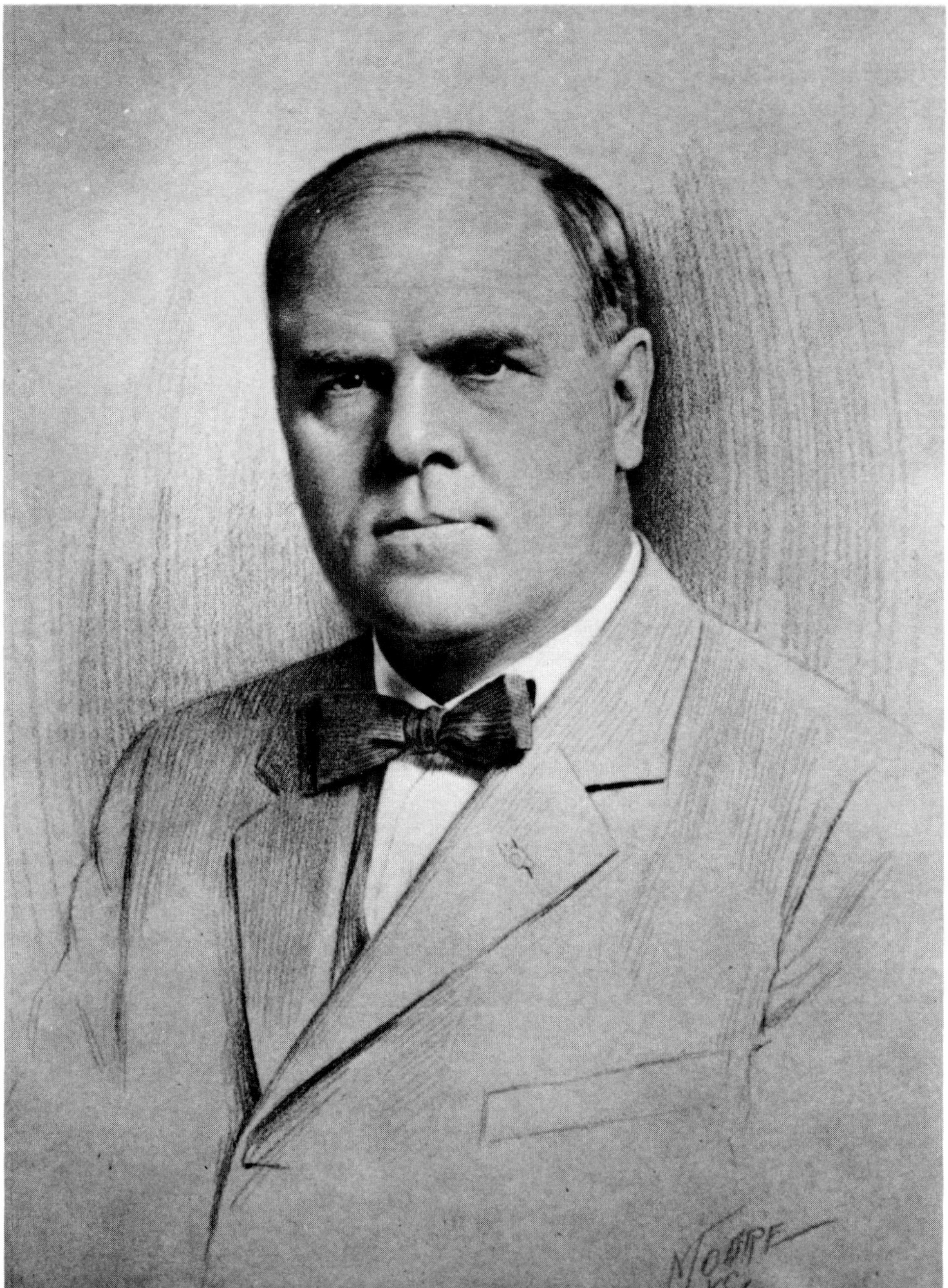

**RICHARD L. SUTTON**
**July 9, 1878—May 18, 1952**

*(From a portrait made in 1925.)*

# Biography

SUTTON, RICHARD LIGHTBURN, dermatologist; b. Rock Port, Mo., July 9, 1878; s. John Grant and Virginia (Robertson) S.; student U. of Mo., 1898-99; M.D., Univ. Med. Coll., Kansas City, Mo., 1901; student Med. Dept. Geo. Washington U., 1903-04, M.D.; U.S. Naval Med. Sch., 1904; grad. study, Johns Hopkins Med. Sch., and in London, Hamburg, Berlin, Vienna and Paris; LL.D., U. of Mo., 1922; hon. Sc.D., Washburn College, Topeka, Kan., 1925; m. Lena Igel, January 3, 1906; children—Richard Lightburn, Emma Louise (Mrs. Lewis H. Moore). Asst. surgeon, U.S. Navy (retired); formerly prof. dermatology, U. of Kan., now prof. emeritus; spl. rep. dept. of natural history, U. of Mo., African expdn., 1923-24, and expdns. for same dept. to Indo-China and India, 1925-26; headed African-Asiatic expdn., 1929-30, Arctic expdn., north of Spitsbergen, as spl. rep. dept. of natural history, U. of Kan., 1932; expdns. to New Zealand and Australia, investigating habits of swordfish, 1935, 36, 37, 38, 39, 40, Peru, 1941; with East Arctic Patrol, Northwest Territories, to Ellesmere Island, Somerset Island and Baffinland, summer of 1939. Trustee Kansas City Museum. Served as pvt. 4th Mo. Volunteer Infantry, Spanish Am. War. Mem. bd. dirs. Salvation Army Kansas City, Mo. Corr. mem. Swedish Dermatological Society, 1950. Life fellow Royal Geographical Society, 1924; Fellow Royal Soc., Edinburgh, 1925; mem. A.M.A. (chmn. dermatol. sect., 1913-14), Jackson County Med. Soc. (pres. 1913-14), Am. Dermatol. Assn., French Geog. Soc., Alpha Kappa Kappa, Med. Library (pres. 1917-19); corr. mem. British Dermatol. Soc.; hon. mem. Southwest Clin. Assn. Mason (32°). Clubs: American Polar Society (New York); Aransas Pass Light Tackle, Tampico Tarpon, San Pedro Marlin; Bay of Islands, Swordfish and Mako Shark Club (Russell, N.Z.); Tauranga Angler's (Bay of Plenty, N.Z.); Bermagui Big Game Anglers' (Australia); New South Wales' Rod Fishers' Soc. (hon.). Author: An African Holiday, 1924; Tiger Trails in Southern Asia, 1926; The Long Trek, Around the World with Camera and Rifle, 1930; Diseases of the Skin (10th edit., with Richard L. Sutton, Jr.), 1939; An Introduction to Dermatology (4th edit., with Richard L. Sutton, Jr.), 1941; Synopsis of Diseases of Skin (with Richard L. Sutton, Jr.), 1942; An Arctic Safari, 1932; The Silver Kings of Aransas Pass and Other Stories, 1937; A Handbook of Dermatology (with R. L. Sutton, Jr.), 1949, part 2, 1950; sect. on The Mycoses in Tice's System, 1919, rewritten (with R. L. Sutton, Jr.), 1940; Collected Verse, 1946, also numerous sci. articles in Am. and fgn. jours. Contrb. to lay periodicals. Home: McAllen, Tex. Deceased May 18, 1952; ashes interred Forest Hill Cemetery, Kansas City, Missouri.

From *Who's Who in America,* Marquis Company, with permission; amended.

## Richard Lightburn Sutton, M.D., Sc.D., LL.D.

DR RICHARD L. SUTTON died on May 18, 1952, at the age of seventy-three years, from coronary thrombosis following an operation for diaphragmatic hernia. He was one of the ten children of John Grant and Virginia Robertson Sutton of Rock Port, Missouri, and spent his youthful years on the farm of his father, who, an early settler from Kentucky, was a minister of the Campbellite Disciples of Christ. All the daughters were school teachers and all the sons earned medical degrees.

Richard Sutton's dreams in the time of his childhood were of travel, exploration and adventure. His mind was curious and brilliantly clear. His thought processes were lightning-fast. His perception of the feelings and motives of his fellows was quick and sensitive. His emotions were demonstrative. His body was strong and big. His vigour and exuberance were amazing throughout his life to all who knew him. His communicativeness, vivacity and ability to evoke warmth and affection were such that it was said of him, "He made friends while other people wasted time". His pockets and the drawers of his desk were filled with trinkets for children. He had in the highest degree the capacity to make a person feel better through the effulgence of his own vitality and the impress of his hearty voice and handshake. Where he was, people knew it and were happier.

He taught school at Rock Port for a time, then volunteered in 1898 in the Missouri Infantry in the Spanish American War. This lasted but a few months, during which he showed his lifetime interest in people and observation by writing letters to the home-town newspaper. There followed medical schooling at the University Medical College of Kansas City, Missouri, where he won the $100 gold prize for highest scholastic standing on graduation in 1901.

Further education included not only an association with Dr P. G. Unna of Hamburg, Germany, but also a *locum tenens* for a country doctor in a Kansas village, and studies at Johns Hopkins, London, Berlin, Paris, and the United States Naval Medical School. He said, however, that the vast proportion of what he learned "he dug out for himself the hard way"—possibly that is the chief way by which an original mind learns. He served briefly as a Lieutenant (j.g.) in the United States Naval Medical Department, from which he was separated in 1905.

Dr Sutton married Lena Igel of Leavenworth, Kansas, in 1906, and they made a permanent home in Kansas City, Missouri, where he practised dermatology until his retirement in 1940. There are two children, Richard

L. Sutton, Jr., M.D., born in 1908, of Kansas City, Missouri, and Emma Louisa Sutton Moore, born in 1914, of McAllen, Texas, who, with his widow living now also in McAllen, survive him.

Dr Sutton was active in medical society affairs, being President of the Jackson County, Missouri, Medical Society, and also Chairman of the Dermatologic Section of the American Medical Association in 1913. He gave the original descriptions of Periadenitis mucosa necrotica recurrens (*Journal of Cutaneous Diseases* 29: 65, 1911) and Leukoderma acquisitum centrifugum (*Journal of Cutaneous Diseases* 34: 794, 1916), the latter being known in medical dictionaries as "Sutton's Disease". The first edition of his classic text, *Diseases of the Skin*, published by C. V. Mosby Company, St Louis, Missouri, appeared with 915 pages and 693 illustrations in 1916 (which was the year his mother died), and subsequent editions were almost biennial. The tenth edition, in 1939, in collaboration with his son, contained 1549 pages, 1452 illustrations, and a bibliography of approximately 30,000 entries.

He lived a life of "do it now": when a new edition was in preparation, he continued to manage an office practice of from 200 to 250 patients per day, and wrote from after supper until one or two o'clock in the morning for a period of three or four months until the job was done. He interspersed during his medical career numerous expeditions to far corners of the earth, often as a representative of some museum, fetching home specimens, collections, photographs and notes which he enthusiastically transformed into short stories and books on travel.

Dr Sutton's character as a citizen, a traveller, a hunter and fisherman, a writer, and a productive scientist is attested by his generosity to the Penny Ice Fund of the Salvation Army; his donations to the Kansas City Museum and to the natural history museums of the Universities of Kansas and Missouri; his gifts to the Kansas City Zoo of animals brought back from various travels; his Professorship of Dermatology at the University of Kansas Medical School for a period of some thirty years; his contribution to Kansas City, Missouri, of funds providing for a wading pool in a park for Negro children; his expeditions to Africa, India, Indo-China, Spitsbergen, New Zealand and elsewhere; his authorship of many articles and several books on dermatologic subjects, and of books on travel (*An African Holiday*, *Tiger Trails in Southern Asia*, *The Long Trek*, *An Arctic Safari*), and of numerous short stories which appeared in such magazines as *Outdoor Life*, *Field and Stream*, and *The American Rifleman* (collected in a volume entitled *Silver Kings of Aransas Pass*); his memberships in the American Polar Society, the Royal Geographical Society of London, the Port Aransas Light Tackle Club, the Tampico

Tarpon Club, the Bay of Islands Swordfish and Mako Shark Club, the Tauranga Angler's Club, the Bermagui Big Game Angler's Club, the New South Wales Rod Fishers' Society, and the American Dermatological Association; and his honorary degrees of Doctor of Laws from his University of Missouri Alma Mater and Doctor of Science from Washburn College. He was elected a Fellow in 1925. He collected autographed and association volumes. His library contained a great many books of poetry, which he appreciated and of which he wrote a little.

After his son joined him in the practice of medicine, Dr and Mrs Sutton together visited the big game fishing waters of Australia, New Zealand, Nova Scotia, Tampico, and elsewhere frequently and with delightful comradeship. The war years brought these trips to an end, and, when wars were largely over, failing health precluded strenuous enterprises. In 1946 they moved their residence to McAllen, Texas, to escape rigorous winters and to enjoy the company of their daughter and her sons. During the last years he fought valiantly, with never-failing buoyancy, zest for life and optimism, for the sense of well-being which had been his habit, and he endured in a period of two years six major surgical endeavours. Throughout these bad times, which eventuated in his death, he expected to get well and again to go fishing, for he loved to fish; and he possessed the devotion of his courageous wife and a multitude of friends from all walks of life.

RICHARD L. SUTTON, JR.

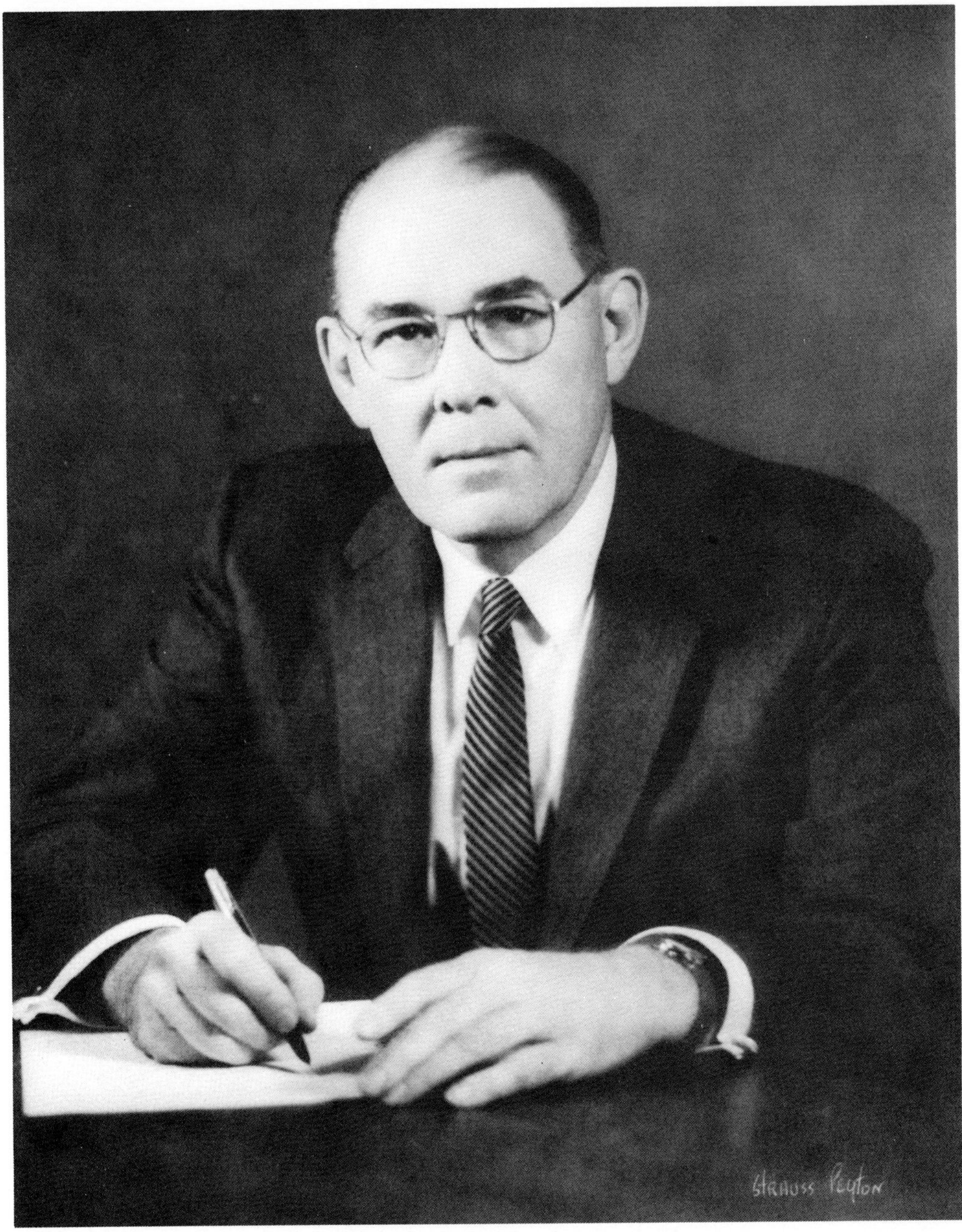


RICHARD L. SUTTON, JR.

*(1962)*

# Biography

SUTTON, RICHARD LIGHTBURN, JR., physician; born in Kansas City, Missouri, May 11, 1908; son of Richard L. and Magdalena Schussler Igel S.; Country Day School for Boys (Kansas City, Missouri) 1916-1923; B.S. University of Michigan, Ann Arbor, 1927, A.M. (in Embryology under G. Carl Huber) 1929, M.D., 1929; Licentiate Royal College of Physicians and Surgeons, Edinburgh, Scotland, 1932. Internship Cleveland City Hospital 1930-31 (under Harold N. Cole). Postgraduate study Royal Infirmary, Edinburgh (under Sir Norman Walker). Preceptorship approved by American Board of Dermatology & Syphilology under Richard L. Sutton, Sr., 1933-1940; certified by Board, 1937.

Married Serena Anne Neel, September 28, 1935; children: Serena Lee (Mrs. Dean E. Tollefson), Richard Neel, M.D., diagnostic radiologist; Anne Louise (Canfield), journalist; Elizabeth Ellison (Mrs. Michael Benefiel).

Began career in the practice of dermatology in 1932 as employee of Richard L. Sutton, Sr., who retired in 1940. Consultant Ellis Fischel State Cancer Hospital, Columbia, Missouri. Associate in dermatology, University of Kansas 1932-35, assistant professor 1939-46, associate professor 1946-49, professor, chairman of department 1949-56, clinical professor of medicine (dermatology) 1956-1969, clinical professor emeritus 1969. Research associate Paleontological Institute, University of Kansas, 1966-1973. Clinical professor of medicine University of Missouri Medical Center 1967-70; senior consulting professor University of Missouri—Columbia. Adjunct professor of geosciences University of Missouri—Kansas City, 1970-. Established UMKC Geology Museum (with Prof. Eldon Parizek) opened to public November 1973, D.Sc. (honorary) UMKC 1975. Instr. chemical warfare 1942; consultant Dermatoses Investigation Sect. USPHS (under Louis Schwartz) 1942-49. Chief, section of skin and syphilis (US Army neurosyphilis center) Woodrow Wilson General Hospital, Staunton, Virginia 1943-45; senior consultant in dermatology Veterans Administration. Served from captain to major MC AUS 1943-46. Diplomate National Board Medical Examiners (1929); Conjoint Board of Medical Examiners of Scotland (1932); American Board Dermatology and Syphilology (1937). Fellow A.M.A., A.A.A.S., Royal Society (Edinburgh), Royal Geographical Society (London). Member American Dermatological Association (elected 1940, v.p. 1969-70), Paleontological Society, Polish Dermatological Society (hon.), Southern Medical Association (hon.), Jackson County (Missouri) Medical Society (hon.), Johnson County (Kansas) Medical Society (hon.); Heart of America Geology Club (pres. 1963,

1973), Austrian (hon.), Venezuelan (hon.) dermatological societies. Phi Delta Theta, Phi Rho Sigma, Phi Sigma, Alpha Omega Alpha, Sigma Xi. Member Jackson County (Missouri) Historical Society. Trustee The Barstow School 1955-1958 (pres. 1957-58).

Afro-Asiatic expedition 1929-1930 with Richard L. Sutton, photography and collection of big game in Tanganyika (Tanzania) and French Indo-China (Vietnam) for University of Missouri-Columbia and Dyche Museum, University of Kansas (see Sutton, Sr. *The Long Trek,* 1930; Jr. contrib. chapters on Mbulu ethnology and Swahili language). Spitsbergen expedition with Richard L. Sutton summer of 1932 collecting polar bear, walrus, seal and bird specimens for Dyche Museum (see Sutton, Sr. *An Arctic Safari,* 1933). Legally blind 1976 (macular degeneration). Donated collection on billiards to International Sports Library, Notre Dame University (1977). Designed and published with Melissa Duffner, B.F.A., "Low Vision 20/200 Playing Cards," 1980. Cofounder with Drs. Felix Sabates and John Irvine, Low Vision Clinic, Truman Medical Center, Kansas City, Missouri (1981). Adjunct Professor in Ophthalmology, University of Missouri School of Medicine, Kansas City, Missouri, 1980-. See also, J. Am. Acad. Dermat., Dec. 1981.

Home: 3203 West 83rd Terrace, Leawood, Kansas 66206.

From *Who's Who in America,* Marquis Company, with permission; amended.